Praise for *The Doctor-Approved Cannabis Handbook*

"As a cancer survivor and a cannabis advocate, I know the important medical role cannabis can play. Dr. Caplan's new book offers a wealth of information and a huge dose of compassion and clarity."

—Melissa Etheridge

"As the owner of the first medical cannabis dispensary on the East Coast, I understand the importance and effectiveness of cannabis therapies. *The Doctor-Approved Cannabis Handbook* is the first comprehensive medical guide that provides groundbreaking new solutions to many of the medical issues that affect us all, including anxiety, sleeplessness, and pain management."

—Howard Kessler, entrepreneur and philanthropist, and founder and owner of New England Treatment Access (NETA), the first East Coast medical marijuana dispensary

"*The Doctor-Approved Cannabis Handbook* is an authoritative compilation of cannabis-based therapies, ideal for anyone considering an effective, safer alternative to many mainstream traditional therapies. Dr. Caplan's thorough research, thoughtful analysis, and practical guidance leave you with hope that you will feel better, and a deeper appreciation of the many ways that cannabis positively interacts with the human body."

—William Van Faasen, former chairman and CEO of Blue Cross Blue Shield of Massachusetts, and director of Acreage Holdings, a national cannabis investment company

"The biggest barrier currently preventing millions of people from realizing the potentially life changing benefits of medical cannabis is the lack of clinical engagement and support. Dr. Caplan's extensive experience as one of the country's leading medical cannabis practitioners and researchers makes a compelling case that cannabis treatments combined with clinical guidance can help patients realize the full benefits of a medical marijuana regimen and understand the risks of DIY treatment. Patients and physicians seeking and providing treatment can effectively reduce symptoms from a wide range of conditions with limited side effects."

—Steven J. Hoffman, inaugural chairman of the Massachusetts Cannabis Control Commission

"Dr. Caplan is one of the most experienced healthcare providers when it comes to the medicinal usage of cannabis. Given the longstanding federal research restrictions on cannabis and the lack of cannabis education in medical school, there are only a few individuals like Dr. Caplan who are at the leading edge of the field. *The Doctor-Approved Cannabis Handbook* is a wealth of knowledge resulting from Dr. Caplan integrating what official research is available with his tremendous clinical experience treating countless patients with medical cannabis."

—Jeff Chen, MD, cofounder and CEO of Radicle Science, and founder and former director of the UCLA Center for Cannabis and Cannabinoids

"In the seminal legal case in America regarding medical cannabis, NORML vs. DEA, the chief administrative judge of the DEA in 1988 ruled, 'Marijuana, in its natural form, is one of the safest therapeutically active substances known to man.' Thirty-five years later, Dr. Benjamin Caplan affirms such in his comprehensive and scholarly work."

—Allen St. Pierre, former executive director of the National Organization for the Reform of Marijuana Laws (NORML)

"*The Doctor-Approved Cannabis Handbook* provides a clinically oriented and approachable translation of often complex and confusing data regarding cannabis medicine. Caplan builds on the many thousands of patients that he has helped over the years and highlights the therapeutic options for those who are interested in considering the use of cannabis-containing products."

—Harvey J. Berger, MD, founder, former chairman, and CEO of ARIAD Pharmaceuticals, Inc., and former executive chairman of Medinol, Inc.

"Dr. Caplan's extensive clinical experience provides the reader with a comprehensive understanding of how medical cannabis can be used to improve health outcomes."

—Caroline A. MacCallum, MD, leading cannabis clinician, researcher, and educator

"Dr. Benjamin Caplan's *The Doctor-Approved Cannabis Handbook* is a comprehensive and informative guide to the potential benefits of cannabis for a variety of medical conditions, general health and well-being, and end-of-life care. Dr. Caplan is a highly-trained, well-respected physician and researcher, and has done an excellent job of distilling the complex science of cannabis into a clear and concise guide. The book is a treasure of information that patients, their families, and physicians can learn and benefit from, with key insights on the different types of cannabis products, and how to use cannabis safely and effectively."

—Karyemaître Aliffe, MD

"I have found the information contained in Dr. Caplan's book to be extremely useful, and it has helped me in many ways, including better sleep, better attitude, [and] happier days. I strongly endorse his book."

—Michael Berns, PhD

The Doctor-Approved Cannabis Handbook

The
DOCTOR-APPROVED
Cannabis
Handbook

Reverse Disease, Treat Pain, and
Enhance Your Wellness with
Medical Marijuana and CBD

BENJAMIN CAPLAN, MD

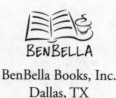

BENBELLA

BenBella Books, Inc.
Dallas, TX

BenBella Books, Inc.
10440 N. Central Expressway
Suite 800
Dallas, TX 75231
benbellabooks.com
Send feedback to feedback@benbellabooks.com

BenBella is a federally registered trademark.

Printed in the United States of America
10 9 8 7 6 5 4 3 2 1

Library of Congress Control Number: 2023015031
ISBN 9781637742679 (trade paperback)
ISBN 9781637742686 (electronic)

Editing by Scott Calamar
Copyediting by Michael Fedison
Proofreading by Sarah Vostok and Marissa Wold Uhrina
Indexing by WordCo.
Text design and composition by PerfecType, Nashville, TN
Cover design by Brigid Pearson
Printed by Lake Book Manufacturing

This book is dedicated to my parents, Brenda and Lou, the greatest healthcare duo I know. For eight decades, they have tirelessly cared for others with compassion and love, and have inspired me to do the same. This book is written with endless gratitude for your unwavering commitment to making a positive impact in the world.

Contents

Introduction

The world is changing its opinion of "cannabis as medicine," and you are the beneficiary of this revolution. Not ten years ago, the majority of traditional doctors wouldn't dream of prescribing cannabis to their patients, insisting that it was dangerous and unstudied. Yet once their patients began sharing the positive outcomes they were discovering, and the relief they were experiencing, doctors slowly began the shift toward a "don't ask, don't tell" policy. This small level of acceptance was an important first step, but in reality, it wasn't all that helpful to their patients. We turn to doctors when we need specific health advice, and this attitude was anything but specific.

Today, a second shift toward greater understanding and acceptance is taking place. Many of the most conservative medical practitioners from the finest hospitals are recommending that their patients consider medical cannabis, at times even before other traditional medicines. Over the past ten years, the scientific press has been publishing more cannabis research than at any other time in history. At the same time, the public outcry for legalization of cannabis paved the way for normalizing cannabis therapies. Growing communities of cannabis enthusiasts have also coalesced to spread information and education about the effectiveness of cannabis treatments. A true scientific understanding now shows that there is a diverse set of medical concerns and symptoms that cannabis can address.

With this level of normalization, you may be able to finally address your mental or physical concerns with a legitimate and effective strategy. There is a clear path to easy, safe, and legal access to medical and/or adult-use (twenty-one and over) cannabis products that can meet your needs. And you will likely find that many of your friends and family are also benefiting from these treatments already. According to a recently published study in *JAMA* (the *Journal of the American Medical Association*), marijuana use has risen year over year among people over sixty-five since 2015.[1]

Cannabis products offer a complete pharmacy of benefits, from anti-inflammation to pain relief, muscle relaxation to sleep assistance, mood disorder support to reversing weight gain or loss. In fact, cannabis can help relieve many of the symptoms related to the major chronic illnesses that adults face. That's why I put this book together. In this one resource, you will be able to address your ailments by accessing the most relevant cannabis recommendations for treatments. With my guidance, you will be able to formulate treatment protocols with nuance and variety so that you can find better solutions and achieve outcomes that are perfect just for you. While it may take a little time to determine the best dosing and product match, many of my patients are thrilled that they can enhance, and eventually replace, many of their current medications.

Cannabis Upends the Treatment Protocol Model

I often call guided cannabis medicine a "choose your own adventure" model, because the wide range of products is itself a completely different approach to medicine. In the past, you would have gone to a doctor to address a specific illness. The doctor would write a prescription for a specific medicine, which would either help you—or not. Traditional treatment decisions are based on *population-based medicine*: the results of high-quality research, including randomized control trials that arrive at conclusions reached by studying the average experience of lots of different people. Your doctor used that data to prescribe you a medication based on your explanation of how you felt during that single office visit, rather than having good access to your daily living experiences at home. If the first treatment didn't work, you came back, and the doctor would give you a different prescription.

The problem is, that data and that type of medical practice actually never applied to any one person, nor anyone's real-life circumstances. The result is that your prescription—the type of drug you took, its frequency, and amount—was based on what was best for a whole group of people, and not what was known to be best for just you.

Guided cannabis therapies tip that model on its head and offer an appealing new option, not only because of the medicinal properties of cannabis, but because of the sense of empowerment you will achieve. You can be in control of what you consume, how much you consume, how often you consume, and how you consume. You will have the option to adapt your program, or what I call *self-titrate*, on days that you need more, or cut back when you need less. And, you can choose different products to elicit different effects. For instance, you can choose among properties that will suppress your appetite, or ones that will increase it.

Best of all, cannabis doesn't have the side effects or the potential risk profiles of traditional pharmaceuticals. Unlike the "diarrhea or death" litany of side effects often mentioned on pharmaceutical commercials on TV, the most common downsides of cannabis might be initial sleepiness, temporary light-headedness, or an increase in appetite. What's more, the usual fears about prescription medications interacting in harmful ways with other prescriptions are rarely a concern when you introduce cannabis.

Welcome to a Whole New Way of Looking at Medicine

With the multitude of treatment options that cannabis brings to the table right now, the relationship between the patient and the physician completely changes. Doctors like me are acting more like a trusted resource who makes individualized suggestions from an expert's point of view instead of playing the role of a commander who delivers generic prescriptions and hopes for best outcomes. The truth is, the old model of the omnipotent doctor is broken, and we know this because patients are not getting better. Too many people are told that they have to "learn to live" with the "aches and pains of life" instead of eradicating them. I wouldn't want to live with the constant agony of pain or illness, and neither should you. And while many well-intentioned doctors want to offer guidance based on the best available evidence, the rate at which the science is changing is staggering, and too many doctors continue to practice with out-of-date information.

The latest science confirms what I've found to be true: that cannabis may, in fact, be the secret sauce for those who have been down the traditional medical road before and have come up short in terms of resolving their health complaints. So many of my patients have struggled excessively and unnecessarily with therapies that simply never worked for their bodies or their schedule. Just as some people respond to certain medicines better than others, many people respond to cannabis therapies who didn't respond well to other options.

Cannabis products seem to be much better suited to meeting patients where they are, supporting them now while leaving room for adjustments over time. Enlightened doctors can have deep discussions with their patients to find out where each person is coming from, what their personal experience is, and what their health goals are. With that specific knowledge, we can guide patients to the right products, the right dosages, and at the same time, give them the latitude to experiment and arrive at the personalization they are looking for.

Welcome to My Guided Cannabis Medical Practice

Right now, there are a plethora of cannabis products that can resolve a host of medical problems, yet a paucity of doctors focusing on the medical guidance model. My aim is to deliver that connection by providing you with an authoritative and practical understanding of the many uses and benefits of cannabis medical treatments so that you can resolve your own health problems. You can also take this book to your doctor. Show them that there is a new way of looking at medicine and new options to explore. Then together, we can help you get you to a better, healthier place.

I am a licensed, registered, board-certified family physician. In 2012, I started working with telehealth patients and turned my family medicine practice to one that is known throughout the world as a preeminent cannabis practice. I have overseen the medical guidance of cannabis care for more than 250,000 people. In short, I provide cannabis care as if it were already a medical specialty.

Before then, I was not exactly the poster child of pot smokers. The truth is, I didn't know anything about cannabis. I grew up with the same misguidance, misinformation, and ignorance around cannabis that all of us had heard. During my teen years, I was warned by well-intentioned folks, including my family and my doctors, that marijuana was a gateway to maladaptive coping strategies or drugs that would cause harm, if not kill me. I took that message to heart, because nobody I personally knew who was reputable or intelligent consumed cannabis (at least openly).

I followed my father into the family business, which was medicine. When I got to medical school in 2006, I was never taught anything of substance about cannabis, despite the growing cultural acceptance of its therapeutic effects. Instead, my earlier impressions of cannabis were solidified because in medical school it was taught only through the lens of addiction, dependence, and maladaptation. Sadly, that lack of clinical education that could support new physicians in training remains, even today.

I focused my medical education on the goal of having a family medicine practice. I would treat all kinds of people who suffer from a wide range of illnesses, and I liked the challenge of trying to develop expertise in many different subjects: I could be a psychiatrist with one patient, a rheumatologist with another, and a dermatologist later in the day. This model also suited my idea of what an ideal physician should be. I decided early on that I would stay at the forefront of medicine, listen carefully to my patients, and encourage them to be open with me. My primary goal was never to pass pills, but to help my patients consider their own best options.

Over the years, there were times inside my clinic when my patients felt comfortable enough to be completely open, whether it was about their drug use, their sexuality, or their relationships. It was through these candid conversations that my patients first introduced the medical benefits of cannabis to me. This oral tradition is a theme for cannabis in our culture: even in the face of political, social, cultural, or spiritual adversity, cannabis use survives because its effects are told from one person to another. As I was charting these particular patients' health progress, I was astounded by how well they were doing: their health was improving, they appeared happier and less physically and emotionally burdened by their illnesses, and often, they were able to give up other prescription medications, over time.

I decided that the best way to help my patients with this unfamiliar terrain was to completely immerse myself in the research so that I could then relay it in a way that was intelligible and digestible. I started reading everything I could get my hands on about cannabis: the positive, the negative, and the agnostic. Over the years, I built my knowledge base, and by 2015, I was deeply familiar with the accepted peer-reviewed medical literature. While there were some clinical studies that reported positively about patient experiences, the vast majority continued with the prevailing negative campaign. That was no surprise, as most of the medical literature available at that time was patient-related cannabis research funded by the National Institute on Drug Abuse. However, I was reading enough that I saw glimpses of possibilities. I realized that the gold standard of scientific studies—randomized control trials—is not ideal for monitoring the effects of guided cannabis, because the placebo effect itself is governed by the same system in the brain that reacts to cannabis use (you'll learn more about that later in the book). And more importantly, I realized that what I was seeing in my own clinic didn't match what the studies were showing.

I set out to create my own data set of user experiences to codify the clinical results I was witnessing. I began to interview doctors across the country where medical marijuana was legalized. And when it became legal in Massachusetts, where I practice, I put out my shingle as a physician who specializes in medical cannabis. I knew that many of my peers judged me. They saw me as a sellout, and they couldn't believe that cannabis therapies were a legitimate path in medicine. But I was undeterred.

Through my work guiding thousands of patients, I have had the privilege of learning from their successes and failures with cannabis. Through their journeys and their willingness to document their treatments, I have been able to create an authoritative longitudinal data set related to guided clinical cannabis outcomes and best practices. By poring over this data, I can offer each new patient who comes to see me a pathway to healing based on the lessons learned from others. And the results have been nothing short of amazing for the range of symptoms and conditions that are covered in this book.

My strategy is to work with each patient and recommend a specific starting point to meet their needs, and then follow up at regular intervals to see how these suggestions are working, making modifications along the way that reflect the realities of the patients' lives and improvements in their health. I typically start my patients conservatively with doses that are generally not euphoric and amounts that are not overwhelming, not impactful in daily life, not changing someone's usual experience, and then increase gradually until they're feeling comfortable. This is the same methodology you will be able to use by following the guidance in this book. The truth is, nobody really knows what your optimal dosage of any medication should be, or which products will be the most effective.

Today, I'm involved with all aspects of cannabis medicine. I am a clinician who works with patients. I am also a researcher who is contributing to the scientific literature, including an article published in the *New England Journal of Medicine*. I have found that one step better than randomized, evidence-based science is mathematical fact, and that comes from discerning polling. If we poll enough people on their experience with guided cannabis medicine, including details about themselves, the products they choose, and the circumstances when they take them, we can approach a mathematical certainty in terms of best practices. In effect, I'm doing my own crowdsourcing. Along with my own patients, I have formed a company that is creating the largest clinical data set about cannabis consumption. In fact, you can join along and share your experience. By downloading the EO Care app on your smartphone, you will be able to participate in this data collection. Your feedback on your experience will help create an educated platform that is not only improving your own care, but also helping others.

I'm also an advocate, working to raise awareness, share my knowledge, and bring new, effective products to market. As you'll learn, there's more to cannabis than THC and CBD: there's a cornucopia of other molecules in the cannabis plant that should be made more readily available. (While it's easy to get many of the most basic products, some of the more medicinally beneficial properties remain hard to find in the marketplace, so I will teach you how to make what you need at home: more on that later, too.)

Lastly, I've had the privilege of collaborating with Howard Kessler, who almost single-handedly created the credit card industry we know today. Howard's passion matches my own for helping people address the normal ailments of aging that are neglected by modern medicine. Our vision is a complete restructuring of the national approach to medical cannabis. He's coordinating private/public partnerships for cannabis-based therapies between senior care businesses and the US government toward creating broad, national acceptance. There aren't many people who could do that, and to have the privilege of playing an educational role in that discussion is a tremendous honor for me to complete my mission.

All of this is to say that you've come to the right place. While I'm very familiar with a wide range of cannabis resources, be assured that you've chosen the most authoritative voice in the field. No other website, book, or podcast will match the range and scientific knowledge found in this book. Dispensary agents might have personal experience with cannabis but no formal medical education. Pharmacists are just beginning to become well versed in the literature, but as of this writing there are only nine states that enable pharmacists to serve as educators and dispensers of product: Arkansas, Connecticut, Minnesota, New York, Pennsylvania, Louisiana, Utah, New Hampshire, and Maryland. Instead, you will benefit from my formal medical training, my extensive research, and my clinical experience treating thousands of patients with cannabis, so that you can address your specific needs.

How This Book Works

If you've never used cannabis/marijuana/weed, welcome! I'm going to be right here with you now as you ease your way into these new therapeutic options. And if you have tried cannabis in the past, get ready for a whole new experience. Modern cannabis and its related products are much more suitable to a variety of users and uses than what you may have come across in the past. If you like its euphoric effects, there will be many, many options for you to try; and if you were scared of it in the past, there are products that omit that experience entirely.

Part I provides a comprehensive overview of the cannabis plant, how it affects your health, and the plant's different properties that we can take advantage of. For instance, some cannabis products can be used to reverse disease; others can address and manage the often uncomfortable symptoms that occur during the disease process. Many people also experience its benefits as a ripple effect, addressing multiple brain and body complaints simultaneously. With that understanding, you will learn how and where to purchase a wide variety of products, and create ones at home to meet your individual needs.

In Part II, you will see how cannabis can be integrated into a personalized treatment protocol. Medical conditions are organized in broad terms and are easy to find within each of the chapters. You will gain a better understanding of your illness or condition, the related signs and symptoms, and the potentials for cannabis to be a solution. You'll also learn why traditional medicine may not have worked ideally in the past, and you'll follow some of my patients to find out how they effectively used these treatments. The broad categories covered include:

+ Mental health
+ Insomnia
+ Headaches
+ Dementia, Alzheimer's disease, and Parkinson's disease
+ Seizures
+ Pain
+ Gastrological issues
+ Skin conditions
+ Sexual health
+ Cancer
+ End of life

I've observed that people who don't find success with cannabis are few and far between. All you really need is a sense of curiosity and a little bit of patience. Combined with the right guidance and first-rate products, your quality of life and sense of well-being will improve along with your health.

Are you ready to ditch the pain, improve your mood, or just get a good night's sleep? The possibilities for not just good health, but great health, start right here. Let's go!

PART ONE

A Guided Cannabis Overview

CHAPTER 1

The Cannabis Plant

Whether or not you are new to cannabis, cannabis use is certainly not new. In fact, the cannabis plant has been a part of human life for tens of thousands of years, which is one reason why it might be an ideal match as a medicine for us. Cannabis is a complex plant that naturally contains an entire pharmacy of therapeutic compounds. The better you understand the cannabis plant and its therapeutic components, the easier it will be to identify the right properties and the right products to meet your particular health needs.

Our ancestors evolved alongside the cannabis plant and literally cultivated a symbiotic relationship along the way—just as panda bears evolved to fulfill their nutritious needs with bamboo, monarch butterflies coevolved with milkweed, and koalas became symbiotic with eucalyptus. In fact, there is a historical treasure trove of documented experience that connects this plant directly to human ancestors. Archeological evidence of cannabis harks back 12,000 years,[1] yet the first record of its use in medicine dates back to the world's oldest written recording of medicinal drugs, the Chinese *Sheng-nung Pen-ts'ao Ching*, compiled in the first century AD. In the US, Dr. William Brooke O'Shaughnessy first wrote about the medicinal aspects of cannabis in 1839, and it was recognized in the *United States Pharmacopeia* as a legitimate medical compound in 1851.[2]

Cannabis cultivation and consumption spread quickly throughout the world, as it is a plant that is easy to grow and is incredibly adaptive. It can grow in arid locations just as easily as fertile ones. More importantly, the plant itself changes with its environment. It adjusts its growth patterns to optimize exposure to light, rain, and soil quality, as well as the time of year it blooms, and to what array of aromatic compounds it produces when it blooms. Like fine wines, the assortment of environmental conditions influences a specific terroir, resulting in a wide range of plant characteristics. This is why some cannabis products smell like fresh mint and pine, and others like lavender or skunk.

Over the centuries, farmers learned that the cannabis plant was useful in many ways and could be cultivated to get the most useful properties out of it: from increasing the euphoric experience to strengthening the plant's fibers so that it could be used for rope, paper, or thread. As each different use was identified, and farming techniques improved to optimize certain characteristics, the plant evolved into several distinct gene pools. While similar in appearance, the varieties of genders/relatives are, at the same time, starkly different in their growth product. Some gene pools of the female cannabis plants produced bigger flowers that create lots of potentially smokable stuff and contain large amounts of the compound THC. Taller, stronger, and more fibrous plants that were easier to harvest were singled out for industrial use: these plants became known as hemp. It just so happens that the hemp plants that produce a lot of fiber and small flowers contain fewer compounds that produce a euphoric, intoxicating effect, and the genetic relatives of those plants happen to produce CBD. This natural duality of cannabis presents two families of choice that you will be learning about in this book. In fact, these families existed as far back as six hundred years ago, when manual laborers were making paper, roof thatching, and rope out of hemp by day, and then smoking its cousin for its medicinal effects.

Yet the cannabis plant offers much more than strength and psychedelics. Because of its environmental adaptability, the cannabis plant developed a full range of chemical diversity. Many of its chemical components and/or compounds were used as powerful medicines for thousands of years, with a wide range of applications. As time went on and farming techniques improved, the characteristics that were highly prized were cultivated, and the ones that seemed less relevant for the market were bred out and became nearly obsolete. Today, almost 95 percent of the original chemical components previously found in cannabis have been drastically reduced.

However, not all is literally lost. While certain components may be diminished, they are not forgotten. Inside the leaves and flowers of the current relatives of both of these plant families are hundreds of already-identified compounds that can be activated to provide tremendous medicinal value. All we have to do is identify, learn about, and access them.

First, let's look more closely at the plant and understand the full range of opportunities it offers. That's the guidance part of guided medical cannabis: the scientific evaluation of these different components.

The Origin of *Marijuana*

I prefer the word *cannabis* to almost all terms used to describe this plant, including pot, weed, bud, ganja, hemp, kush, reefer, and marijuana. This last, and probably the most popular, term does in fact carry a racist connotation.

The addition of *marijuana* to the lexicon starts out innocently enough. It's a Spanish word that came from Mexico, and was brought to the US when legal Mexican immigrants were fleeing the Mexican Revolution in the early twentieth century. US prohibitionists who were spreading their fears that cannabis was making people crazy, stupid, and silly, and anti-immigration advocates who were mocking Mexicans as lazy and incompetent, seemingly combined their efforts and quickly adopted the term to use it in a derogatory way, emphasizing the relationship with the plant's hallucinogenic effects and Mexican migrants.

While the word *marijuana* is regularly used around the world, for legislative initiatives, and in everyday speech, it's not scientific and does not represent the medicinal qualities discussed in this book. Until we can totally erase it from the common parlance, we can try to take one small step to make this world a better place, stamp out racism whenever we see it, and purposefully choose *cannabis*: a name that gives scientific validity and stature to this healing plant. In fact, the industry standard uses the word *cannabis* to describe both the plant itself and the products derived from it.

Basic Botany: Cannabis Plants

The cannabis plant has developed in different parts of the world from three separate gene pools: *sativa* (tall with narrow leaves), *indica* (short with wide leaves), and *ruderalis* (the shortest with sparse leaves). These subtle differences have little relevance now when it comes to buying products.

You may be familiar with the terms *cannabis* and *hemp* and think that they are from different plants. In actuality, they are from the same cannabis plant species. Every cannabis plant is comprised of a stalk, leaves, seeds, and flowers (buds). There is a male plant and a female plant, with the female producing flowers and seeds. Across a variety of well-established industries, and over millennia, every part of the plant has spawned its own commercialized use, to some extent.

+ The main stem, or stalk, grows straight from the root system. It is used for textile fibers. The male and female stalks are used to produce a spectrum of products, from soft material used for clothing, to stronger fibers used in rope.

+ The leaves contain some useful pharmaceuticals (about 8 percent). There are fan leaves, which are the larger, easily identifiable leaves. Sugar leaves are small, resin-coated leaves that protect the flower, or buds. These can be used for extracts and other cannabis chemical compound products.

+ Cannabis seeds are a perfect match for human nutrition. They contain fiber, protein, minerals, carbohydrates, and even the good fats like the omega-6 and omega-3. Interestingly, cannabis seeds contain these compounds in the precise proportions that mirror human nutritional requirement ratios.

✦ Flowers contain the vast majority of the chemical compounds used, and
are where most of the medicinal value of the plant is pulled from. The
cola, or *bud site,* is the name for a cluster of flowers growing together. Each
flower is coated with *trichomes,* a clear resin secreted from the glands of the
plant. Trichomes contain the aromatic oils that give the plant a variety of
scents, and are where both THC and CBD are harvested from.

The Chemical Components of Cannabis

Scientists have identified roughly six hundred different chemical compounds
among the various types of cannabis plants. And over the last several decades,
researchers have begun to uncover what effects each of these compounds has on
our health. For instance, some compounds increase inflammation, while others
decrease it. Some can put a pause on cancer cell reproduction, while others have
evidence of being cardioprotective or improve the body's processing of sugar.

These compounds are grouped as either cannabinoids, terpenes, or flavonoids.
Each group is chemically different from the other, but they all functionally share
many similarities. Many people think that cannabinoids are the only compounds
that matter, but as you'll see, that simply isn't true. The fact is, cannabis medicine
offers so much more when you understand how all of the compounds work independently and in synchrony.

Defining Euphoria

Euphoria refers to the altered state that is some combination of relaxation,
joy, peacefulness, and contentment. There are levels of each of these feelings that can be achieved depending on one's biology, mood, personality,
dosage, and type of cannabis ingested. With so many factors, the euphoric
experience will be different for everyone and can even be different under specific circumstances within one individual's experience.

Over time, people have summarized this complex state with one oversim-
plistic term: *being high.* It's not my favorite, because it carries the connotation of

an experience that is unpredictable and out of one's control. Instead, I prefer the term *euphoria* to connote an experience that is attainable with guided cannabis therapies featuring THC products: it is replicable, controllable, and therapeutic.

So, *euphoric* is used in conjunction with products that contain THC; *non-euphoric* is used for CBD products. You may also run across terms like *psychoactive*, *intoxicating*, and *inebriating*, which are often used in cannabis culture to describe THC effects. *Psychoactive* in particular is an overused and overly general term that applies to anything that affects your thinking and feeling. For instance, the act of splashing cold water on your face to invigorate you could be called psychoactive, as well as a lemon-scented, warmed hand towel applied to the face. For their diverse effects on the brain, all cannabis products can be considered psychoactive. Even though CBD does not create a euphoric effect, taken at the right dosage, it will have direct effects on your state of mind while not seeming to affect your mental clarity.

Cannabinoids

Cannabinoids are the molecules synthetized in the trichomes of female flowers. They interact with the plant's environment, shielding its reproductive parts from ultraviolet light (so that they aren't damaged), and they interact with other plants and animal life so that the cannabis plant will thrive, naturally attracting and repelling certain wildlife.

Cannabinoids are the molecules that bind to, activate, inhibit, or otherwise influence the actions of cannabinoid receptors and the associated signaling pathways in the brain and body to release a specific effect. We are all born with cannabinoid receptors, which can be found in almost every cell of the body. Usually, these receptors are kept busy with our inherently manufactured cannabinoid molecules. That's right: we already have cannabinoids inside our body, and you'll learn more about that in the next chapter. When an additional group of plant-derived compounds, which look and act almost identically to those we already have, interact with the body's receptors, impactful changes and reactions arise.

The Cannabinoid All-Stars: THC and CBD

The two most abundant cannabinoids are *tetrahydrocannabinol*, known as THC (or more specifically, Delta-9 THC), and *cannabidiol*, or CBD. CBD is most prominently found in the more fibrous, stocky male plant (hemp). The female plant also produces CBD in its flower, but because it is mixed with many other cannabinoid components, it is less prevalent and therefore less efficient to collect.

CBD and THC have different medical benefits, as well as many overlapping ones. Often, either can provide relief for several of the same conditions. The reason is that on a microscopic level, the shape and chemical makeup of these two molecules is nearly indistinguishable. They so closely mirror one another that they differ in only one subcomponent. This subtle difference in molecular shape, however, bears tremendous impact on how these two molecules interact with receptors in the body, yielding starkly different effect sensations.

The difference most commonly recognized is that CBD products won't cause the euphoric effects that occur with THC products, yet they are often just as effective for the same conditions/symptoms. Unfortunately, THC has developed a bad reputation, and in my opinion it is undeserved. It has been cast away from modern appreciation and medicinal care while CBD has been embraced as having merit and value. This is in large part because the US government has given a public seal of approval to CBD while continuing to shun THC as having "no medicinal value" and keeping its status as a Schedule I substance.

Out of a misunderstanding of the negligible differences between the chemical makeup of these two compounds, two similar industries evolved, with very different regulatory structures, and because of this single difference, the US federal and state governments have established two distinct, multibillion-dollar legal markets. The THC market is very highly regulated. The CBD market is starting to be self-regulated (not by the government). Rigorous testing is a requirement in the THC-based industry, while CBD product manufacturers turn to third parties for testing and can share that information with the public, although they are not mandated to do so. This difference in regulation is why some complain that CBD products are a scam or don't work.

These two compounds can work either individually or in synchrony. If the consumed cannabis consists of a uniformly homogenous volume of THC molecules (called an *isolate*), the activation of the body's cannabinoid receptors is more aggressive, and typically, you will feel the effect more intensely. With its subtle differences in shape, however, CBD consumed at the same time can act as a buffer to THC, causing some THC molecules to avoid binding to the receptors, softening the overall response, and occasionally yielding a more favorable therapeutic effect.

Other Cannabinoids You'll Come Across

While THC and CBD are the most well-known and well-studied cannabinoids, they are not the only ones in the cannabis plant that have medicinal properties. Focusing solely on THC and CBD would be like explaining that bread was made from only flour and water; it isn't taking into account the additional ingredients that make certain breads unique, like salt, oil, olives, rosemary, or even nuts.

There are actually more than one hundred unique cannabinoids that have been identified. Some of the most studied include CBG, CBN, Delta-8 (THC), Delta-10 (THC), CBC, and CBDV, each of which have different effects and actions, as well as some that are similar. Yet nearly every chemical compound naturally derived from THC can also be created from CBD. This chemical flexibility creates a confusingly large array of products (some derived from THC, some from CBD) with only subtle clinical differences. Additionally, some compounds simplified with the same name may contain nuanced chemical differences that affect the way they work. For example, THCV derived from THC is more effective than the THCV derived from Delta-8 THC, which is actually derived from CBD. This is important to know because the products you may read about online are not always the same as what you have access to buy. Sometimes, specific products you may have tried in the past have been "improved," or are no longer available at the time you want to purchase them.

And, even though some compounds are sourced from the non-euphoric CBD compound, some of these cannabinoids do have THC-like properties, including degrees of euphoria. For example, Delta-8 THC is produced from hemp, yet its molecular shape is only slightly different than traditional THC (which is scientifically known as Delta-9). Delta-8's euphoric effect is approximately 25 percent of the strength of its Delta-9 sister, but in sufficient amounts, they can feel almost indistinguishable and can cause similar patterns of surprise and discomfort for the unsuspecting (or uninformed) consumer.

The Big Cannabinoid List

The following list features the most recognized cannabinoids and under what circumstances they could be used. I often share this chart with my patients, as it helps them understand what we know right now. However, even though we know that certain cannabinoids work for certain conditions, the market has not delivered products that are higher in one of these lesser-known cannabinoids, outside of a few sporadic outliers, including Delta-8, CBG, and CBN. A remarkable fact is, however, that all of these cannabinoids can be found in many traditional THC and CBD products: to release them at home, you need to bring the product to a specific boiling point (you'll learn how to do this in chapter four).

D9-THC or Tetrahydrocannabinol: This is what most refer to, simply, as THC. It is an anti-inflammatory, appetite stimulant, anti-neoplastic (augments chemotherapy), bowel relaxant, euphoriant, and anti-convulsant that offers neurostimulant relief. It is used to address asthma, cough, glaucoma, insomnia, nausea, pain, muscle spasm, seizure, swelling, multiple sclerosis, diabetes, IBS, and Crohn's disease. When consumed at a high dose, THC is associated with appetite stimulation, paranoia, elevated pulse rate, modulation of the immune system, dry mucous membranes, light-headedness, and sedation.

CBD or Cannabidiol: This is an antidepressant, anti-inflammatory, antioxidant, anti-neoplastic, antipsychotic mood stabilizer. CBD offers strong anxiety relief relative to THC, soothes pain of arthritis, reduces elevated heart rate, improves insomnia, reduces muscle spasm, slows pulse rate, quells nausea and pain, and reduces seizure activity. CBD promotes lipid and blood-sugar level stabilization, promotes immune modulation, and facilitates neuroprotection. Higher doses are associated with a greater effect. CBD can moderate the intensity of effects of other cannabinoids.

CBC or Cannabichromene: This is a cancer-fighting antioxidant. It can function as a strong anti-inflammatory actor addressing pain and swelling, or a 5-alpha reductase inhibitor with sedative, anti-pyretic, anti-mutagenic, and antiviral properties. The compound *CBL Cannabicyclol* is similar and derived from CBC.

CBCA or Cannabichromenic Acid: When consumed unheated (as a tincture or raw flower mixed into something cold, like a smoothie), this is an effective antibacterial, antidepressant, antifungal, anti-inflammatory, anti-neoplastic that is neuroprotective and neuroregenerative. It encourages increased calcium uptake and offers pain relief; it is a sedative, anti-inflammatory agent, and has antidepressant properties. CBCA moderates the effects of THC. When activated by stomach acid or heat, it converts to CBC.

CBDA or Cannabidiolic Acid: When consumed unheated (as a tincture or raw flower mixed into something cold, like a smoothie), CBDA is an antidepressant, anti-inflammatory, anti-neoplastic, antipsychotic that offers relief from anxiety, nausea, pain, seizures, and muscle spasms. It can address hypertension, atherosclerosis, arrythmias, digestion, and stimulates bone growth. It moderates the effects of THC and CBD. When activated by stomach acid or heat, it converts to predominantly CBD, with a smaller portion converted to other CBD derivatives, like CBDV.

CBDV or Cannabidivarin: This is an antioxidant, anti-inflammatory, anti-epileptic, and bone stimulant that also offers relief from nausea and seizures.

CBE or Cannabielsoin: CBE functions as an antidepressant mood stabilizer and anti-tumor agent. When presented with the terpenes linalool or limonene, CBE has sedative- and immunity-boosting properties. Alone it can support relief of anxiety and pain. It can also be a sedative.

CBG or Cannabigerol (converted CBGA): CBG is an antibacterial, antidepressant, antifungal, anti-inflammatory, antimicrobial, anti-neoplastic, bone stimulant, bowel-relaxant (IBS, IBD), and mood stabilizer. It can soothe skin irritations (eczema, psoriasis, acne), reduce anxiety, reverse glaucoma, treat insomnia, address gastrointestinal diseases, and reduce pain.

CBL or Cannabicyclol: CBL is an anti-inflammatory, antibacterial, and anti-emetic that provides relief from chronic pain.

CBN or Cannabinol: This antibacterial, anti-inflammatory, appetite stimulant, neuroprotective euphoriant (mild) also provides relief of ALS symptoms, asthma, nausea, pain, and seizures. It is a sedative that addresses IBS, hypertension, and soothes the skin (eczema, psoriasis, acne). CBN moderates the effects of THC. This product can be derived from either D9-THC or D8-THC with different effects.

Delta-8-THC or Tetrahydrocannabinol: This cannabinoid is an antidepressant, antioxidant, anti-neoplastic, appetite stimulant, neurostimulant, and euphoriant. It's mildly neuroprotective relative to D9-THC, and reduces toxins. It offers relief from anxiety, nausea, glaucoma, insomnia, and pain. Delta-8-THC moderates the effects of THC and is derived from CBD.

THCA or Tetrahydrocannabinolic Acid: When consumed unheated (as a tincture or raw flower mixed into something cold, like a smoothie), THCA is an anti-inflammatory, antioxidant, anti-neoplastic, anti-emetic that improves neural function and offers neuroprotective relief. It can also address arthritis, insomnia, nausea, neurodegenerative diseases, seizures, IBS, and pain. It can moderate the effects of THC. When activated by stomach acid or heat, it converts to THC.

THCV or Tetrahydrocannabivarin: THCV is an antibacterial, appetite suppressant, and euphoriant that is neuroprotective, increases metabolism and short-term memory, and improves speech impairment. It is an anti-convulsant that provides relief from nausea, pain, acne, Parkinson's disease, and seizures. It moderates the effects of THC.

Terpenes

Terpene is a descriptive term used to categorize a particular type of molecular cluster. Terpenes are aromatic compounds found in all plants, and cannabis contains exceptionally high concentrations of them. Interestingly, foods that are high in terpenes are also thought to be healthy for you. For example, the foods featured in a Mediterranean-style diet—olive oil, lemons, red wine—are high in terpenes and thought to be cardioprotective, prevent diabetes, and help keep a consistent weight.[3]

Most of the smells we are familiar with from the natural world—from lemon to cinnamon to pine—are terpenes. Their rich aromas span the gamut: sweet, tangy, citrus sour, woody pungent, and hundreds more. All of these scents can be found in cannabis plants, and where they are grown or what they are grown with will determine which terpenes they contain. What's more, each terpene has a powerful function beyond its scent, driving wellness and enriching the activity of cannabinoid molecules. Some of the common smells of cannabis—fruity, woody, skunky—are terpenes that naturally attract and repel certain wildlife.

The unusual high presence of diverse terpenes is one of the major reasons that cannabis has maintained its popularity (in nature and in human consumption) for millennia. In different regions with different climates, the cannabis plant has adapted to thrive by producing an array of terpenes that optimizes the plant's ability to flourish. For example, in sunny climates, the plant has more terpenes that protect it from harmful UV light exposure; it has also evolutionarily adjusted its composition of terpenes to attract local pollinating insects and repel predators. This innate survival mechanism has meant that it is essentially impossible to find two plants that produce identical chemical profiles. Even within a single plant, the terpene compounds produced at the top of the plant will differ from those at the bottom.

Terpenes have beneficial effects when isolated as well as when they are used in conjunction with cannabinoids. For instance, one terpene called beta-caryophyllene is a molecule that not only has a musky, spicy odor (like cracked pepper), but it also has calming properties. When used at the same time as cannabinoids, either in edible form or in a lotion, the mixture of the two amplifies each compound's effect. This can be useful if you want a pain reliever that will also calm you down.

The Big Terpene List

The following list features the most recognized terpenes and in which circumstances they could be used. Some popular cannabis products already come predisposed to provide specific terpenes, based on the natural plant's growth conditions. Like the secondary cannabinoids, the market has yet to find an effective way to isolate and deliver these ingredients in a consumer-friendly way. It is possible to supplement existing cannabis products so that they are higher in one type of terpene than another by adding terpenes derived from other non-cannabis sources, or by bringing cannabis flower to a specific boiling point (you'll learn how to do this in chapter four).

Cadinene: Anti-cancer, anti-inflammatory, antimicrobial, antiplasmodial. Evidence supports use for treatment of ovarian cancer. Smells like juniper/gin.

Camphene: Antimicrobial, antioxidant, anti-inflammatory, analgesic, antifungal, cardioprotective. Evidence supports use for treatment of fatty liver disease. Smells like turpentine.

Camphor: Analgesic, anti-cancer, antifungal, anti-inflammatory, anti-itch, antiviral, counter-irritant. Evidence supports use for treatment of colon cancer, ovarian cancer, and influenza. Smells sweetly spicy.

Carvacrol: Anti-anxiety, anti-cancer, anti-convulsant, antidepressant, anti-inflammatory, anti-septic, anti-spasmodic, antiviral, gastroprotective, neuroprotective. Evidence supports use for treatment of heartburn, high cholesterol, mouth cancer, gastric cancer, TBI (traumatic brain injury), Parkinson's, stroke, and norovirus. Smells like oregano.

Caryophyllene Oxide: Analgesic, anti-cancer, anti-inflammatory, antioxidant, antiviral. Evidence supports use for treatment of Chagas disease (caused by a parasite), cervical cancer, leukemia, lung cancer, and stomach cancer. Smells like pepper, wood, clove.

Cedrene: Anti-anxiety, hepatoprotective, anti-inflammatory, antifungal, antimicrobial, antibacterial, neuroprotective. Evidence supports use for treatment of anxiety, arthritis, congestion, and hepatic steatosis. Smells like fresh wood.

Cinnamaldehyde: Anti-cancer, anti-inflammatory, anti-platelet aggregating, anti-proliferative, anti-hyperglycemic, anti-hyperlipidemic, neuroprotective, vascular protection. Evidence supports use for treatment of rheumatoid arthritis, lung cancer, atherosclerosis, colon cancer, and Alzheimer's disease. Smells like cinnamon.

Citral: Analgesic, anti-cancer, anti-convulsant, anti-diabetic, anti-inflammatory, anti-parasitic, anti-pyretic, anti-spasmodic, gastroprotective, nephroprotective. Evidence supports use for treatment of skin cancer, lung cancer, breast cancer, rhabdomyosarcoma (a soft-tissue cancer), stomach cancer, fever, and bacterial infections. Smells like lemon.

Citronellal: Antimicrobial, antioxidant, antifungal, anti-cancer. Evidence supports use for treatment of bacterial infections, lung cancer, and breast cancer. Smells like citrus.

Citronellol: Anti-anxiety, anti-cancer, anti-convulsant, anti-diabetic, anti-inflammatory, antimicrobial, anti-spasmodic, chemo-preventive. Evidence supports use for treatment of tachycardia, hypertension, diabetes, cataracts, high cholesterol, and bacterial infections. Smells like lemongrass.

Delta-3-Carene: Anti-inflammatory, antimicrobial, antioxidant, antifungal. Evidence supports use for treatment of cervical cancer, arthritis, osteoporosis, ringworm, and fibromyalgia. Smells sweetly herbal.

Eucalyptol: Analgesic, anti-anxiety, anti-diabetic, anti-inflammatory, anti-spasmodic, antiviral, chemo-preventive, gastroprotective, hepatoprotective, nephroprotective. Evidence supports use for treatment of sinusitis, bronchitis, COPD, influenza, colon cancer, type 2 diabetes, pancreatitis, dyspnea, and hypertension. Smells like menthol.

Eugenol: Anti-cancer, anti-diabetic, anti-inflammatory, anti-parasitic, anti-pyretic, anti-septic, antiviral, cardioprotective, hepatoprotective, neuroprotective. Evidence supports use for treatment of myocardial infarction, hypertension, acute lung injury, leishmaniasis (a parasitic disease), Ebola, HSV 1 and 2, hepatitis, and dermatitis. Smells like clove.

Farnesene: Anti-cancer, antimicrobial, antioxidant, neuroprotective. Evidence supports use for treatment of Alzheimer's disease and Parkinson's disease. Smells like apple.

Fenchol: Antimicrobial, antioxidant, antibacterial, analgesic, anti-inflammatory. Evidence supports use for treating bacterial infections. Smells like basil.

Geraniol: Analgesic, anti-anxiety, anti-cancer, antidepressant, anti-diabetic, anti-parasitic, antiviral, cardioprotective, gastroprotective, neuroprotective. Evidence supports use for treatment of depression, anxiety, Parkinson's, spinal cord injury, IBS, tongue cancer, and endometrial cancer. Smells like fruit, citrus, rose, floral.

Guaiol: Anti-cancer, antimicrobial, anti-parasitic, anti-proliferative, chemo-sensitizing. Evidence supports use for treatment of non–small cell lung cancer and leishmaniasis. Smells like pine and rose.

Humulene: Anti-cancer, anti-inflammatory, antimicrobial, anti-proliferative, chemo-sensitizing, analgesic. Evidence supports use for treatment of breast cancer, colon cancer, lung cancer, and airway allergic inflammation. Smells like hops.

Isoborneol: Analgesic, anti-anxiety, anti-coagulant, antioxidant, anti-parasitic, antiviral, neuroprotective, vasorelaxant. Evidence supports use for treatment of HSV type 1, anxiety, insomnia, Parkinson's disease, hemorrhoids, and leishmaniasis. Smells like camphor.

Isopulegol: Analgesic, anti-anxiety, anti-cancer, anti-convulsant, antioxidant, antiviral, antidepressant, anti-epileptic, gastroprotective. Evidence supports use for treatment of depression, anxiety, liver cancer, epilepsy, and gastric ulcers. Smells like mint.

Laurene: Anti-cancer, antimicrobial, antibacterial, antifungal, antiviral, anti-tumor, anti-ulcer, anti-inflammatory. Evidence supports use for treatment of bacterial infections.

Limonene: Analgesic, anti-anxiety, anti-cancer, antidepressant, anti-diabetic, anti-inflammatory, anti-parasitic, antiviral, chemo-sensitizing, gastroprotective. Evidence supports use for treatment of HSV type 1, kidney cancer, lymphoma, heartburn, Chagas disease, and acute lung injury. Smells like citrus.

Linalool: Analgesic, anti-anxiety, anti-cancer, anti-convulsant, anti-diabetic, anti-inflammatory, antimicrobial, nephroprotective, neuroprotective, spasmolytic. Evidence supports that it is highly calming, and used for treatment of anxiety, epilepsy, allodynia (extreme pain sensitivity), carpal tunnel syndrome, edema, candidiasis, ovarian cancer, and hyperglycemia. Smells like floral, citrus, candy.

Linalyl acetate: Anti-cancer, antidepressant, anti-diabetic, anti-hypertensive, anti-inflammatory, antimicrobial, anti-proliferative, cardioprotective. Evidence supports use for treatment of colon cancer, leukemia, prostate cancer, melanoma edema, and diabetic cardiovascular stress. Smells floral, sweet and citric, minty, and like caraway seeds.

L-Menthol: Analgesic, anti-cancer, anti-inflammatory, antimicrobial, antioxidant, anti-spasmodic, chemo-preventive, cough relief. Evidence supports use for treatment of functional dyspepsia, pancreatitis, anisakiasis (a parasitic disease), respiratory irritation, depression, IBS, and colon cancer. Smells like peppermint.

Longifolene: Antimicrobial, anti-inflammatory, antioxidant, analgesic, anti-spasmodic. Evidence supports use for treatment of breast cancer, menopause, and boosting fertility. Smells woody.

Myrcene: Analgesic, anti-cancer, anti-convulsant, anti-inflammatory, antimicrobial, antioxidant, anti-parasitic. Evidence supports that it is highly calming and used for treatment of bacterial infections, insomnia, and cystic echinococcosis (a parasitic disease). Smells musky.

Nerol: Analgesic, anti-anxiety, antidepressant, anti-inflammatory, antimicrobial, antioxidant, antiviral, cardioprotective, gastroprotective. Evidence supports use for treatment of bacterial infections, ulcerative colitis, and arrhythmia. Smells like roses.

Nerolidol: Anti-anxiety, anti-cancer, anti-convulsant, anti-inflammatory, antimicrobial, antioxidant, anti-parasitic, hepatoprotective, neuroprotective. Evidence supports use for treatment of bacterial infections, leishmaniasis, malaria, schistosomiasis (a parasitic disease), anxiety, Parkinson's, and endometriosis. Smells like wood.

Ocimene: Anti-hypertensive, anti-inflammatory, antimicrobial, antioxidant, antiviral. Evidence supports use for treatment of congestion, bacterial infections, and ringworm. Smells like lime.

Para-Cymene: Analgesic, anti-inflammatory, antimicrobial, antioxidant, gastroprotective, mitigates cholinergic dysfunction (alleviates dryness and promotes better memory). Evidence supports use for treatment of Alzheimer's, Parkinson's, Huntington's, schizophrenia, and gastric ulcers. Smells like wood and turpentine combined with lemon.

Phytol: Anti-anxiety, anti-cancer, anti-cholinesterase, anti-convulsant, antidepressant, anti-diabetic, anti-inflammatory, anti-parasitic, anti-spasmodic, neuroprotective. Evidence supports use for treatment of cervical cancer, neuroblastoma, MS, rheumatoid arthritis, leishmaniasis, malaria, depression, and epilepsy. Smells grassy and floral.

Pulegone: Anti-inflammatory, antimicrobial, antioxidant, anti-anxiety. Evidence supports use for treatment of bacterial infections, congestion, menstrual pain, and atopic dermatitis. Smells like spearmint.

Sabinene: Anti-inflammatory, antimicrobial, antifungal, antioxidant. Evidence supports use for treatment of bacterial infections and bacterial resistance, skin rashes, meningitis, and dental decay prevention. Smells like black pepper.

Terpinolene: Analgesic, anti-cancer, anti-inflammatory, antioxidant, anti-proliferative, antifungal, antimicrobial, anti-anxiety. Evidence supports use for treatment of glioblastoma multiforme (a brain tumor), acute inflammatory diseases, diabetes, Alzheimer's disease, anxiety, and insomnia. Smells floral and herby.

Valencene: Anti-inflammatory, antioxidant, anti-allergic, antibacterial, antifungal, neuroprotective. Evidence supports use for treatment of nail fungus and eczema. Smells like oranges.

α-Bisabolol: Anti-cancer, antimicrobial, anti-spasmodic, cardioprotective, gastroprotective, neuroprotective. Evidence supports use for internal dryness, memory impairment, treatment of stroke, Alzheimer's disease, leukemia, multi-resistant bacterial infections, myocardial infarction, heart failure, hypertension, angina, and ulcers. Smells like chamomile tea.

α-Caryophyllene: Anti-cancer, anti-inflammatory, antimicrobial. Evidence supports use for treatment of bacterial infections.

α-Phellandrene: Analgesic, anti-cancer, antidepressant, anti-inflammatory, antimicrobial, chemo-preventive. Evidence supports use for treatment of depression, rheumatoid arthritis, osteoarthritis, liver cancer, leukemia, hyperalgesia, and breast cancer. Smells herbaceous, woody, minty, and mildly citrus.

α-Pinene: Analgesic, anti-cancer, anti-convulsant, anti-inflammatory, antimicrobial, antioxidant, anti-proliferative, gastroprotective. Evidence supports use for treatment of epilepsy, liver cancer, melanoma, prostate cancer, pancreatitis, osteoarthritis, and asthma. Smells like pine.

α-Terpinene: Antimicrobial, antioxidant, anti-cancer. Evidence supports use for treatment of bacterial infections and breast cancer. Smells like wood and citrus.

α-Terpineol: Anti-cancer, anti-cholinergic, anti-diarrheal, anti-inflammatory, anti-spasmodic, gastroprotective, anti-convulsant, immunostimulant, neuroprotective. Evidence supports use for treatment of bronchitis, gastric lesions, ulcers, breast cancer, lung cancer, brain cancer, epilepsy, and morphine addiction. Smells like peach.

β-Caryophyllene: Anti-anxiety, anti-cancer, anti-convulsant, antidepressant, anti-diabetic, anti-inflammatory, anti-platelet aggregation, hepatoprotective, neuroprotective. Evidence supports use for treatment of Alzheimer's, Parkinson's, MS, alcohol dependence, insulin resistance, melanoma, and endometriosis. Smells like pepper.

β-Pinene: Analgesic, anti-cancer, antidepressant, anti-hypertensive, antimicrobial, antiviral, bronchodilator. Evidence supports use for treatment of HSV type 1, depression, methicillin-resistant Staph aureus (MRSA), and asthma sensitivities. Smells like pine.

β-Terpinene: Anti-inflammatory, antimicrobial, antioxidant. Evidence supports use for treatment of acute inflammatory diseases. Smells like turpentine.

Flavonoids

Flavonoids are another type of compound found in plants that work synergistically and in parallel with cannabinoids to exact powerful medical effects and serve a host of critical medical applications. Like terpenes, flavonoids are a naturally occurring group of plant compounds. While the dietary benefits of certain flavonoids have been known to human cultures for thousands of years (this is why grandparents have been forever telling us to eat fruits, vegetables, teas, red wine, and dark chocolate), the scientific underpinning of their medicinal value is a relatively recent phenomenon. Their value is attributed to both their antioxidative and anti-inflammatory properties, which help stabilize biology that may be prone to mutations such as cancers. One famous flavonoid is resveratrol, which is found in red wine and dark chocolates and is thought to be life-extending.

The Big Flavonoid List

The following list features the most recognized flavonoids and in which circumstances they could be used. Like the secondary cannabinoids, the market has yet to find an effective way to isolate these ingredients. It is possible to source cannabis that is higher in one type of flavonoid than another, but they usually come as part of a THC or CBD product. To release them, you need to bring the product to a specific boiling point (you'll learn how to do this in chapter four).

Acacetin: Anti-cancer, anti-diabetic, anti-hypertensive, anti-inflammatory, anti-parasitic, cardioprotective, hepatoprotective, neuroprotective. Evidence supports use for treatment of acute lung injury, atrial fibrillation, breast cancer, diabetes, malaria, and ulcerative colitis.

Alpinetin: Antibacterial, anti-hemostatic, antioxidative, anti-hepatotoxic, immunosuppressive, anti-inflammatory. Increases appetite and digestion. Evidence supports use for ulcerative colitis, acute kidney injury, and endometritis.

Amentoflavone: Antioxidant.

Apigenin: Anti-anxiety, anti-cancer, anti-cholinesterase, anti-diabetic, anti-dyslipidemic, anti-inflammatory, antiviral, hepatoprotective, neuroprotective. Evidence supports use for adenovirus, African swine fever virus, Alzheimer's, breast cancer, hepatitis B, irritable bowel disorder, and lupus.

Apiin: Antibacterial, antifungal, antioxidant, hepatoprotective, anti-diabetic, analgesic, spasmolytic, immunosuppressant, anti-platelet, gastroprotective.

Arbutin: Evidence supports use for lower urinary tract infection, cystitis, kidney stones, and as a diuretic.

Astragalin: Anti-inflammatory, antioxidant, neuroprotective, cardioprotective, anti-obesity, anti-osteoporotic, anti-cancer, anti-ulcer, anti-diabetic.

Azaleatin: Antioxidant, anti-inflammatory.

Baicalein: Anti-amyloidogenic, anti-cancer, anti-convulsant, antidepressant, anti-diabetic, anti-fibrogenic, antiviral, cardioprotective, hepatoprotective, neuroprotective. Evidence supports use for acute liver failure, asthma, bladder cancer, cardiac hypertrophy, dengue fever, epilepsy, gout, hepatic fibrosis, and HIV.

Baicalin: Anti-inflammatory. Evidence supports use for irritable bowel disorder.

Bilobetin: Neuroprotective.

Butin: Antioxidant, anti-platelet, anti-inflammatory. Evidence supports use for myocardial infarction, to improve heart function, and diabetes-induced cardiac oxidative damage prevention.

Cannflavin A: Antioxidant, anti-parasitic. Evidence supports use for leishmaniasis.

Cannflavin B: Antimicrobial, anti-parasitic. Evidence supports use for leishmaniasis.

Catechin: Antioxidant, anti-cancer.

Chrysin: Anti-cancer, anti-inflammatory, neuroprotective. Evidence supports use for irritable bowel disorder.

Daidzein: Anti-inflammatory. Evidence supports use for irritable bowel disorder.

Delphinidin: Anti-proliferative, cardioprotective. Evidence supports use for atherosclerosis.

Diosmetin: Anti-cancer, anti-diabetic. Evidence supports use for liver cancer and diabetes.

Diosmin: Anti-cholinesterase, anti-diabetic, anti-dyslipidemic. Evidence supports use for Alzheimer's disease and type 2 diabetes.

Epicatechin: Neuroprotective.

Epigallocatechin gallate: Anti-inflammatory, antioxidant, cardioprotective, chemo-preventive, hepatoprotective, neuroprotective. Evidence supports use for adrenal cancer, atherosclerosis, bladder cancer, cervical cancer, irritable bowel disorder, osteoporosis, and steatohepatitis.

Eriodictyol: Anti-inflammatory, anti-allergenic (helps prevent the development of allergies), antimicrobial, anti-cancer, and antioxidant. Evidence supports use for retinal inflammation.

Fisetin: Anti-inflammatory, antioxidant, anti-proliferative, cardioprotective, neuroprotective.

Fustin: Anti-hyperglycemic, antioxidant, antimicrobial, anti-arthritic, anti-obesity, anti-platelet, and anti-cancer.

Galangin: Antiviral, anti-inflammatory, anti-diabetic, antioxidant, and anti-cancer. Evidence supports use for irritable bowel syndrome (IBS) and asthma.

Genistein: Anti-allergy, anti-atherogenic (alleviates arterial plaque growth), anti-cancer, anti-fibrotic, anti-hypertensive, anti-thrombotic, antiviral, chemo-sensitizing, neuroprotective. Evidence supports use for asthma, brain edema, cardiac fibrosis, HIV, insulin resistance, lymphoma, and metabolic syndrome.

Genistin: Anti-cancer, anti-inflammatory.

Genkwanin: Anti-cancer. Evidence supports use for breast cancer.

Geraldol: Antioxidant, anti-inflammatory, and mitigates new blood vessel growth.

Ginkgetin: Anti-inflammatory. Evidence supports use for chronic skin inflammation and cerebral ischemia/reperfusion (lack of blood flow in stroke/healing of stroke) injury.

Glabridin: Anti-inflammatory. Evidence supports use for irritable bowel disorder.

Glycitein: Antioxidant. Evidence supports use for postmenopausal osteoporosis, type 2 diabetes, and breast cancer.

Glycitin: Anti-osteoporotic. Evidence supports use for bone loss prevention.

Gossypetin: Anti-amyloidogenic. Evidence supports use for Alzheimer's disease.

Hesperetin: Anti-inflammatory, antioxidant, antiviral. Evidence supports use for high cholesterol, high lipids, and neuroinflammatory injury.

Hesperidin: Anti-allergic, anti-cancer, anti-convulsant, antidepressant, anti-diabetic, anti-proliferative, antiviral, cardioprotective, neuroprotective. Evidence supports use for asthma, colitis, diabetic retinopathy, Huntington's disease, ischemic heart disease, and multiple sclerosis.

Homoeriodictyol: Antioxidant, antibacterial, limits cancer mutations. Evidence supports use for osteoporosis, breast cancer, cervical cancer, colon adenocarcinoma, and bacterial infections like *staphylococcus aureus*, *salmonella typhi*.

Ipriflavone: Anti-allergic. Evidence supports use for milk allergy, peanut allergy.

Isoginkgetin: Anti-cancer, anti-diabetic, anti-inflammatory, antioxidant, anti-radiation, anti-thrombotic, chemo-sensitizing, neuroprotective.

Isoliquiritigenin: Antioxidant, anti-inflammatory, antiviral, anti-diabetic, anti-spasmodic, and anti-tumor. Evidence supports use for psoriasis.

Isoorientin: Hepatoprotective.

Isoquercetin: Antioxidant, anti-thrombotic. Evidence supports use for prevention of thrombus formation.

Isorhamnetin: Anti-cancer, anti-fibrotic, anti-inflammatory, limits the reproduction of cancer cells, anti-thrombotic, antiviral, cardioprotective, hepatoprotective, neuroprotective. Evidence supports use for acute inflammatory diseases, bacterial sepsis, cardiac hypertrophy, gastric cancer, heart failure, and influenza.

Isosakuranetin: Antibacterial, antioxidant, anti-protozoal.

Isovitexin: Hepatoprotective.

Kaempferide: Anti-carcinogenic, anti-inflammatory, antioxidant, anti-hypertensive, antibacterial, and antiviral. Evidence supports use for pancreatic cancer prevention.

Kaempferol: Analgesic, antidepressant, promotes the degradation of bones, anti-proliferative, antiviral, bronchodilator, cardioprotective, hepatoprotective, insulin sensitizing. Evidence supports use for alcoholic liver injury, anaphylaxis, bacterial resistance, bone cancer, encephalomyelitis, fibrosarcoma, and HSV.

Linoleamide: Anti-cancer. Evidence supports use for breast cancer.

Luteolin: Anti-allergic, anti-cancer, anti-cholinesterase, anti-diabetic, anti-inflammatory, antioxidant, anti-proliferative, cardioprotective, hepatoprotective, nephroprotective. Evidence supports use for acute myocardial infarction, alcoholic liver disease, atherosclerosis, cataracts, colon cancer, traumatic brain injury, and Alzheimer's disease.

Mangiferin: Hepatoprotective.

Maysin: Anti-obesity. Evidence supports use for weight loss.

Morin: Neuroprotective, anti-inflammatory. Evidence supports use for Alzheimer's disease.

Myricetin: Anti-amyloidogenic, anti-hyperlipidemic (excessive fat deposits in blood), anti-thrombotic, antiviral, cardioprotective, chemo-preventive, hepatoprotective, neuroprotective. Evidence supports use for acute kidney disease, arrythmia, colon cancer, glaucoma, hepatic steatosis, ischemia, liver fibrosis, and multiple sclerosis.

Myricitrin: Anti-inflammatory, antioxidant, anti-carcinogenic, and neuroprotective. Evidence supports use for diabetic nephropathy.

Naringenin: Anti-atherogenic, anti-atherosclerotic, anti-convulsant, anti-diarrheal, anti-fibrotic, anti-mutagenic, anti-thrombotic, anti-ulcer, antiviral. Evidence supports use for arthritis, cardiorenal syndrome, colitis, dyslipidemia, epilepsy, gestational diabetes, IBS, and ischemic stroke.

Narirutin: Anti-allergic, anti-inflammatory, antioxidant. Evidence supports use for asthma, atopic dermatitis, Alzheimer's disease, alcoholic liver disease, inflammatory diseases, and myocardial infarction.

Ononin: Anti-inflammatory, neuroprotective.

Orientin: Hepatoprotective.

Patuletin: Anti-arthritic, anti-cancer, anti-inflammatory, antimicrobial, pain relief, antioxidant, anti-proliferative, anti-spasmodic, antiviral. Evidence supports use for breast cancer, hypertension, influenza, and rheumatoid arthritis.

Phloretin: Antioxidant, anti-cancer, anti-inflammatory, glucose-transporter inhibitor. Evidence supports use for osteoporosis, cancer, diabetes, and obesity.

Phloridzin: Antioxidant, anti-diabetic, anti-hyperglycemic, anti-hyperlipidemic. Evidence supports use for fever, malaria, postprandial hyperglycemia (in diabetes) and diabetes.

Pinocembrin: Anti-fibrotic, anti-inflammatory, antimicrobial, antioxidant, anti-tumor, hepatoprotective, neuroprotective, vasodilator. Evidence supports use for Alzheimer's disease, cerebral ischemia, melanoma, and Parkinson's disease.

Poncirin: Anti-tumor, anti-diabetic, antibacterial. Evidence supports use for asthma, bone loss, inflammation, colitis, gastric cancer, gastritis, liver injury, and Alzheimer's disease.

Quercetagetin: Anti-cancer, anti-diabetic, anti-inflammatory, antimicrobial, antioxidant, anti-proliferative, antiviral. Evidence supports use for diabetes, hepatitis C.

Quercetin: Anti-amyloidogenic, anti-anxiety, anti-cancer, antidepressant, anti-mutagenic, anti-septic, anti-thrombotic, antiviral, cardioprotective, insulin-sensitizing. Evidence supports use for allergic airway inflammation, breast cancer, glioma, heat stroke, HSV, hyperglycemia, IBS, lung cancer, and myeloma.

Quercitrin: Anti-inflammatory. Evidence supports use for irritable bowel syndrome.

Rhamnazin: Anti-neoplastic, antioxidant.

Rhamnetin: Metabolite, antioxidant, anti-inflammatory. Evidence supports use for hepatocellular carcinoma and chemotherapy sensitizing.

Robinetin: Antioxidant.

Robinin: Anti-inflammatory. Evidence supports use for arthritis.

Rutin: Anti-inflammatory, antioxidant, hepatoprotective. Evidence supports use for colitis.

Sakuranin: Antioxidant, anti-inflammatory, anti-cancer, anti-tumor. Evidence supports use for cancer, osteoarthritis, and osteoporosis.

Sciadopitysin: Antioxidant, vasoactive. Evidence supports use for bone fractures, osteoporosis, and osteopenia.

Scopoletin: Anti-hepatotoxic, antibacterial, antifungal, anti-tubercular, and antioxidant. Evidence supports use for headache and rhinitis.

Scutellarein: Antioxidant. Evidence supports use for cerebral infarction and ischemic stroke.

Silibinin: Anti-allergy, anti-cancer, anti-cholinesterase, anti-inflammatory, antimicrobial, antioxidant, neuroprotective. Evidence supports use for Alzheimer's disease and drug-resistant mycobacteria.

Silymarin: Anti-cancer, anti-inflammatory, antimicrobial, antioxidant, antiviral, hepatoprotective. Evidence supports use for hepatic carcinoma and hepatitis C.

Sitagliptin: Anti-diabetic, antioxidant, neuroprotective. Evidence supports use for Alzheimer's disease, epilepsy, and type 2 diabetes.

Spinacetin: Anti-cancer, anti-inflammatory. Evidence supports use for prostate cancer.

Tangeretin: Anti-inflammatory, antioxidant, gastroprotective, neuroprotective. Evidence supports use for Alzheimer's disease and Parkinson's disease.

Theaflavin: Antioxidant, antiviral, anti-cancer. Evidence supports use for high cholesterol, heart disease, and cancer.

How a Plant Becomes a Product

The cannabis products that you will be buying likely come from plants grown in idealized environments of quality-controlled levels of air, water, and nutrients. When the timing is right, the plants are harvested, and the parts that are not richly dense in the active compounds we've discussed are removed. The plants are treated with either supercooled carbon dioxide or frozen butane, neither of which bind to the chemistry of the compounds (although some people mistakenly believe they do). The kief, or the plant parts that are rich in cannabinoids, terpenes, and flavonoids, crack off and fall into a catch-basin, and are then further processed in this concentrated form. Kief can be pressed into many different sticky forms, which you'll learn about in chapter three.

The kief contains the full spectrum of compounds, which is known in the marketplace as "whole plant" or "broad spectrum" cannabis. The individual compounds within kief can also be further separated in a laboratory by their molecular weight differences, or through a heat selection process whereby the plant's molecules are separated into individual components. Alternatively, individual components can also be separated when they are subjected to specific pressures inside a vacuum container. In this way, THC can be separated from CBD, and terpenes and flavonoids can be further extracted as desired.

A Typical Cannabis Experience

It's very important to understand that the cannabis and cannabis products you will be interacting with are vastly different from the pot you or others around you may have smoked years ago. In fact, if you haven't tried it lately, the products that are available today in stores, dispensaries, and on the street are both more potent and more purified. One reason is that when people talk about weed of old, they're literally talking about old weed.

Going as far back as the 1950s to as late as the 1970s, cannabis was either homegrown and not very well cared for, or it was grown in Central and South America, and then shipped across the US. Back then, illegal drug trafficking wasn't known as a superior business model, and it took a long time to get from grower to customer. As cannabis ages, it actually changes chemically, and the percentage of active THC and nutritional terpenes and flavonoids diminishes and changes, not unlike how a banana changes flavors and colors as it ages. With age, the sensory and beneficial effects of the cannabis diminished considerably. For many, those changes may have made the consumed product more appealing than what is available today.

Beginning in the 1980s, the percentage of THC within each plant was bred to be much stronger: in some strains it even doubled. Yesteryear's cannabis used to contain between 8 percent and 15 percent THC; today it's quite common for there to be more than 21–30 percent THC. What's more, as local plant growth has become more feasible and socially accepted, fresh terpenes and regionally unique flavonoid content have similarly developed and improved. Whereas cannabis may have once been full of prominence and noteworthy sensory effects (stinky), it has since become an overflowing factory of nutritional terpene and flavonoid abundance.

Today, cannabis is brought to market in a fresher, more robust state because it can be legally grown in many states across the US. As a consequence, it has a different chemical profile, and depending upon the method of delivery (fresh flower, solutions of cannabinoids dissolved in oils, cooked edibles, etc.), its inherent chemical profiles are now amenable to new combinations with other popular agents (melatonin, caffeine, wine, antioxidants, etc.). What's more, legally purchased modern cannabis is subject to rigorous testing and safety standards in order to reach a completely new level of purity.

As you've learned, the natural chemical variability within each cannabis plant was once multifactorial and diverse. However, the growing demand from consumers of particular attributes means that producers only focus on the specific factors that satisfy the marketplace. The naturally self-moderated makeup of the plant has long been bred out, in favor of powerful plants that can produce the desired ingredients. Much like the way Olympic athletes train in one domain to be the world's best, plants are often bred to excel at producing solely a high-quality THC or CBD.

Later you'll learn how to choose products that have the compounds that will address your symptoms and conditions. You will also learn how to maximize the effectiveness by combining available products and using them in specific ways. As more people like you become fully educated and demand begets supply, the cannabis industry will be incentivized to cultivate a wider range of plants for each of these properties. In the not-too-distant future, you will be able to purchase products that have been created to contain specific high concentrations of cannabis-related terpenes and flavonoids. As it is today, the market offers some products that contain numerous amounts of one or another terpene, generally speaking, but almost always targeted with smell or taste goals in mind, not their physical or psychological impact.

There are already significant advantages to the products that you will be interacting with. A legal, established market allows for uniformity: you can expect the same results every time you have an edible from the same brand. You will also have complete information on what's included in these products: the components that you want to consume, so you can feel confident that it's free of components that you don't want to consume. Overall, this means that the products are safer and more predictable, even if they may be stronger. For medical conditions that are amenable to relief with cannabis, having a reliable product that offers a consistent benefit is a tremendous advantage.

What's Next

In the next chapter you'll build on your plant knowledge to learn how cannabis in general, and these compounds specifically, interact with the body and brain to achieve better health outcomes.

CHAPTER 2

How Cannabis Works

From the time of the shamans, people looked to the plant world for answers. The vestiges of that worldview still exist in our life: we drink coffee when we're sluggish, or pop a mint when we have digestive distress. We also know that people on every continent have used the cannabis plant throughout human history as a regular part of life, and often to provide relief. There are archeological and historical records of cannabis use for medicinal purposes across thousands of years, covering areas from China to India to Africa to South America, and eventually to the US.

The earliest settlers in the Jamestown colonies grew cannabis and used it both medicinally and for currency. By 1839, physicians like William O'Shaughnessy were providing cannabis extracts to patients for its analgesic and sedative properties.[1] The peak of cannabis use as medicine in the US was during the early twentieth century, when it could be easily obtained as an over-the-counter remedy, and there were more than a hundred scientific papers published on its therapeutic use.[2]

By the 1930s, cannabis use was on the rise for both recreational use and medication. Police and government officials pushed for new restrictive legislation. Even though the American Medical Association continued to support its use, in 1937, the Marijuana Tax Act took effect, putting a prohibitive tax on those who grew the plant, and subsequently squelched the entire market. By 1941, all medicinal uses were erased from the American pharmacopeia, and investigations toward its beneficial uses did not begin again until 1964 when the molecular structure of THC was discovered. In 1970, cannabis was considered a Schedule I substance under the federal Controlled Substances Act, and officially classified as to be without medicinal value.

In spite of the wide-ranging efforts to cast cannabis as a cultural taboo, knowledgeable, vocal advocates for the plant have remained powerful. Beginning in earnest after 1988 when the endocannabinoid system was first discovered, medical research in cannabis is more prolific than ever before. Today, cannabis use has come full circle. Against generations of headwinds and all likelihood, the majority of public opinion once again supports comfortable access to the therapeutic benefits of cannabis for those who want it.

The Endocannabinoid System in Action

Cannabis can uniquely influence both the brain and body, which makes it an ideal therapy for so many areas of health. The reason: it has the ability to communicate with just about every cell in the body via *the endocannabinoid system*. *Endo* refers to molecules that are produced inside your body. *Cannabinoid* refers to the collection of molecules and their precursors—either naturally occurring within the body, or produced from plants—and their receptors in the body. This receptor/molecule combination activates a massive array of positive health effects. Cannabis products are literal copycats of endocannabinoids: they are almost identical to the form and function of the naturally occurring molecules that are found in almost all living creatures.

The endocannabinoid molecules we naturally produce are called *anandamide (AEA)* and *2-arachidonoylglyerol (2-AG)*. AEA is found in nearly all animal tissues and some plant tissues. 2-AG is found at high levels in the nervous system, and is derived from the same essential pathways as AEA. There are also cannabinoid molecules that are produced outside of the body, specifically from plants, which are called *phytocannabinoids*. All plant-derived cannabis products, whether they are THC-based or CBD-based, are considered phytocannabinoids.

As endocannabinoids are so prevalently produced throughout the body, scientists believe that the purpose of the system is to maintain overall balance, or *homeostasis*, and keep our internal functions running smoothly. We know that the system impacts mood, memory, appetite, immune function, and nervous system signaling functions. What's more, the endocannabinoid system is a dynamic, evolving ecosystem that adapts to its immediate environment: the body produces and stores endocannabinoid molecules as needed, and these molecules find their way to endocannabinoid receptors in a steady circadian rhythm much like the rhythms of sleep, hormone cycles, fitness, and nutrition.

Whenever we do something that brings us success, we feel a rush of pleasure. In some ways, using cannabis means that we are medicating ourselves with joyful molecules. That response is a manifestation of our body's natural signaling through the endocannabinoid system. When we use cannabis products, the same peacefulness can be re-created from an external tool set that is the same shape and functions as the stuff our body produces naturally, hitting the same receptors.

All types of cannabinoids act as messengers: they send signals to receptors. Almost every cell in the human body has receptors for these molecules, and there are between eighteen and thirty different types of receptors. Whether you are chewing on a cannabis gummy, using a tincture, or applying a lotion, cannabinoids find their way to individual cell receptors. On their way to the receptors, some cannabis molecules go through a *conformational change*, where they are metabolized into different molecules with different interactive properties. Once changed, they can become stronger, while others may become weaker. These molecule changes can allow for binding at different receptors, which may propagate different effects, such as relaxation, increased focus, or appetite stimulation.

Depending on the raw product first consumed, and the strength of your metabolism on a given day, you may have different experiences with the same cannabis. For example, when cannabis is inhaled, the blood vessels may recognize and take in cannabis's raw, unchanged form, which is different from when you consume it orally and it's gone through conformational changes via the gastrointestinal system. Imagine that you tried a candy that is blue in color, which may turn green by the gastrointestinal system as it is digested. If the same amount of cannabis was ingested via inhalation, the body would interpret it as only blue. And if it was a tincture placed under your tongue, the body may see some blue and some green. Someone well hydrated may feel a lighter shade of blue, and someone well rested consuming the product may feel a deeper blue. Such color changes also occur with differences in baseline nutrition, recent meals, metabolism differences, and even hormone cycles. This is the reason why edible products produce longer-lasting effects as compared to inhaled products: the body is seeing a different conformation, which stays around longer.

The cannabinoid's chemical messengers then enter the cells via receptors called *G protein–linked receptors*. These are proteins that cross the cell wall and then create a transcellular communication system to allow for signals to be transmitted from outside to the insides of the cell. Once at the receptors, cannabinoids create effects that are either local (in one area of the body), or systemic (throughout the body). All of our endocannabinoid receptors are waiting to interact with cannabinoid molecules: these molecules are fundamental to influence almost all biological drives, including appetite, memory, temperature regulation, pleasure, pain, and satisfaction.

For example, if cannabis lotion is applied to an arm or a leg, you will have a local response. The reason is that there's a high concentration of cannabinoid and terpenoid molecules, which has a direct effect on local nerves, regional blood vessels, and nearby muscle tissues. You will feel less pain because inflammation is reduced, your muscles will relax where the lotion was applied, or local tumors may shrink and eventually disappear. The lotion molecules will eventually dissipate into the rest of the body, but will not have a strong systemic effect because there aren't enough molecules left to travel through the bloodstream.

If you are using oral cannabis products, you are typically taking a higher dose than what's available in a topical, and there will be enough molecules to spread throughout the whole body. In this case, you are creating a series of local effects everywhere that these molecules travel, acting as multi-location muscle relaxers and system-wide nerve soothers. Systemic products also have indirect effects: you will also experience overall pain relief in each place the cannabinoids are causing local smooth muscle relaxation—it's as if all your cells were saying collectively, "Phew, we are feeling good."

Once the molecules match with a receptor, cannabinoids can influence the body in a few distinct ways. First, they can cause physical changes to cellular walls to allow for enhanced intra- and transcellular communication. This instance of renewed cellular excitement can wake up cells that may otherwise have been dormant. If there is a damaged nerve cell, for example, this spark of life may be enough to kick-start cellular machinery to repair. For inactive stem cells, on the other hand, a cannabinoid jolt at the cell surface might mean rejuvenating the cell's machinery into renewed production mode.

Cannabinoids also have an *epigenetic* effect on cells, or how (and which of) our genes within each cell are turned on or off, which can influence our health. Cannabinoids have the power to increase and decrease the transcription of DNA and the translation of RNA into proteins. They can clean up certain parts of cells to free up dormant actions. For example, in cancer, a cell's ability to self-destruct, called *apoptosis*, is hijacked. One of the ways that cannabis seems to work in killing cancer cells while sparing normal cells is by reinvigorating apoptosis, so that the cancer cells self-destruct and healthy cells are left unaltered.

Cannabinoids can also have a direct effect on nerve signaling, which governs thoughts, movement, and sensory function. You can think about your brain as the top of a pyramid, sending signals down that affect other systems throughout the body via the nervous system. Nerve signals begin as electrical impulses in the brain, and the endocannabinoid system has a powerful effect on this network, causing a slowing down of signaling. That's why when you are using cannabis products, particularly those products that are high in THC, you may feel like you are moving more slowly, and, more importantly, you feel calmer and less hurried.

Cannabinoid molecules mimic some of the natural hormones that our bodies produce. For instance, some cannabinoid molecules have the precise shape to fit into the same receptors to which opiates and narcotics bind. Although the effect of cannabinoids binding the *mu opiate receptors* is only a small fraction of the intensity of opiate medicines bonding there, we still feel slight levity with the cannabinoids without the typical consequences of the addictive narcotics. In fact, many patients who have been prescribed opiates for pain relief end up using far less medication when combined with cannabis products.

Like the ebb and flow of all natural processes, cannabinoids have a life expectancy, and the bloodstream eventually directs cannabinoids to be processed and expelled from the body. Our internal enzymes degrade and dispose of cannabinoids as they process food and other medicines. There are occasionally errors in the degradation system that have fascinating effects and shed light on how the endocannabinoid system functions. For instance, Jo Cameron is a woman who lives in Ireland and is famous because she has no sensation of pain. It turns out that she has a fault with her endocannabinoid destruction enzymes. Rather than being destroyed as they pass through the body, Jo's endocannabinoid molecules continue indefinitely, inoculating her against a stressful life or bouts of physical pain.[3] The downside is that she doesn't have the sensation of pain when it might be helpful. There are also people who don't have the ability to forget, which is another endocannabinoid dysfunction.

Cannabis and the Placebo Effect

We've all heard about *the placebo effect*, where a beneficial result cannot be attributed to the properties of a particular treatment but is due to the patient's belief in that treatment. It turns out that this process may be governed by our endocannabinoid system, and it's especially responsive to cannabinoids brought into the body from outside. Some believe that ingesting just a little bit of extra cannabinoids kick-starts that system to provide dramatic relief.

Cannabis Therapies: The Best Medicine Has to Offer

With this understanding, it's easy to imagine why products made from the cannabis plant do not act like a pharmaceutical drug that targets a single illness, one pathway, or a single receptor; instead, they can provide multifaceted and multipurpose medicine, more like a multi-system therapeutic. In fact, cannabis therapies offer a different, more holistic way of looking at medicine compared to what you may be used to. It is not a pill for an ill formulation, but a total-body approach because it works on the cellular level of every single cell in your body.

Most pharmaceutical medicines and therapies are laser-focused on a single receptor in the body, or provide a single therapeutic molecule or act on a targeted single physiological pathway, in order to treat a specific muscle, organ, or symptom. This hyper-granular focus has habituated modern medicine to disregard the interconnectedness of the multi-system body, and it even influences the way we view disparities and suffering altogether.

Instead, cannabis offers a systemic recalibration that has a global impact in the body: with the right treatment, not only will your pain go away, your experience of pain will also change. My typical patients find a whole new kind of relief, one that's better than what they even have been hoping or searching for. Imagine that the human body is a giant bus that has two drivers: one in the front and another in the back. The medical care we are used to is like having a bus with only one driver: the bus will go forward, but it's not always a comfortable ride. Guided cannabis therapies are like having a bus with two drivers: one who is focused on your emotional state, while the other is managing how the body is healing or feeling. When you leverage both drivers, you have whole-scale healing, delivering a better overall experience, and results that are longer-lasting.

This happens, in part, because, as a fundamental communication molecule, cannabinoids serve as a conduit across two separate body systems. Our bodies are made of separate ecosystems that occasionally interact and respond. For example, your eyes function separately from your nose and your throat, yet if you suffer from seasonal allergies, these separate systems can react simultaneously, warning the rest of the body of possible illness. The endocannabinoid system adds a layer of chemical reinforcement to this inter-system communication. When a cough clears the throat successfully, we feel pleasure at the resulting clarity and comfort, which is the result of the endocannabinoid system functioning. When we believe that we've been given a medicine that will help treat an ailment—the tangible benefit known as the placebo effect—we are also experiencing the benefits of the endocannabinoid system.

Another way to describe how cannabis medicines work is in terms of four factors: peacefulness, comfort, control, and adaptability.

Peacefulness

People who want peacefulness want relief. The mechanism in which cannabis works is very similar to the way the placebo effect works, yet cannabis is not a placebo. The placebo effect is an innate reward system all animals share that helps ensure that their advantageous actions or emotions are continually rewarded. The expectation of a future challenge will be anticipated by the body by flowing stress hormones even before the adversity arrives. Similarly, the benefits of anticipated joys will flow even before the pleasurable event arrives. This autonomously generated physical effect, created by thought and expectation, has real bodily impact. We can re-create that positive response using cannabis.

Buddhism teaches that the ultimate state of meditation is mindfulness, a state of continual presentness. I often describe cannabis as a "tangible essence of meditation," a tool that leverages an organic state of mindfulness. People understand meditation as a dialing back of normal stimulation, normal thought processes, a slowing, a muting of normal input. Just like when we go to sleep and our body and mind slows down, cannabis causes a slowing down of all the body's motors, physically, intellectually, in a way that's similar to meditation. Cannabis softens the control machinery of the mind without disabling it. Rather than rigidly seeking to master one's reality or command control over a condition, an activated endocannabinoid system will deliver relief and a sense of tranquility as it addresses discomfort.

Cannabis can also change one's mental state through its ability to create a momentary sense of forgetfulness. We are so used to the thought trains that are speeding through our mind that we actually depend on them running, even if they're not going in the direction we want to go. When those thought trains carrying our anxieties, discomfort, or anguish are blocked from entering the station via cannabis, we forget about them and experience a new sense of relaxation. In this way cannabis is not only muting your pain signals, it is helping you reframe your relationship with illness.

Let's take post-traumatic stress disorder (PTSD) as an example. PTSD is a syndrome where one experiences an onslaught of memory: you're reliving a particular experience when you are triggered by sensory input. You might think that if you were more present, you would experience more pain, but in essence, it's the reverse. In this case, the desired feature of cannabis is its forgetfulness. Cannabis can help stop those memories from recurring by allowing you to momentarily forget them, which stops the hyper-awareness that leads to feeling jittery. Then the state of mind previously dominated by discontent is replaced by a new state that is better suited to create more agreeable memories.

This experience of peacefulness is entirely within your control: When you are using cannabis therapies, you don't feel drugged. You may feel different from your baseline as your brain slows down, but this change is a temporary effect. It is not going to make you feel dumb or reduce your mental capability. In fact, when you feel more peaceful, calm, and centered, there will be many positive outcomes. You might feel more efficient and productive because you can fully focus on the task at hand. I have patients who report that they can do the work of five people, not just because cannabis is easing their discomfort, but it's actually emptying an overcrowded mind so that helpful, efficient, effective thoughts can have space to form. And by slowing everything down, your own central command gets stronger so that you have more control over what you want to happen on a daily basis.

Comfort

A second positive outcome is an overall sense of mental comfort: of being taken care of. Cannabis is a medicine that positively impacts focus, emotional well-being, and mood, and turns our attention away from things that are unpleasant. Your heart medicine isn't helping you forget about how scary it is to have heart disease, but cannabis may distract you from how depressed you might feel about the disease, or how stressed or anxious or tired you are. In this way, it allows you to continue with your life because you are placing your attention elsewhere. My patient Anna was able to use cannabis to make her physical therapy sessions less emotionally stressful and physically more tolerable. She found that when she uses cannabis, she can better perform the more challenging exercises because her pain is muted and she is more comfortable. This allows her to work just a little bit harder to achieve a better stretch, better extension of her affected muscles, and create a shorter rehabilitation.

Physically, cannabis provides comfort by yielding longer-lasting effects that are less disruptive to everyday life. For example, blood pressure medications might wrench the heart's rhythm lower, and in cases of excess, might cause dramatic effects like fainting, anxiety, and a noticeable cooling of the body. Cannabis's effects are more gradual, which is reassuring in terms of knowing what to expect as it activates in the body.

In many cases, the outcomes of cannabis therapies are better than existing traditional medical treatments. When used either alone or coupled with traditional medicines, cannabis therapies can ameliorate disease processes and make them less severe. Over time, they may replace your existing medication. In my experience, between 50 and 80 percent of people who try cannabis drop at least one other medicine, or reduce the amount they need to control their condition.

Cannabis products can even enhance the effectiveness of traditional medications. For instance, both cannabis and blood thinners like warfarin or Coumadin are broken down in the liver. When taken together, the warfarin is not processed as rapidly, so more of it flows through the bloodstream. This means that some people find that a smaller dosage of warfarin is enough to achieve the same therapeutic effect. And by lowering your dose of warfarin, you may have fewer side effects of that medication, as well as a reduced risk of overdose.

Another reason why cannabis therapies can create more comfort is that compared to traditional pharmaceuticals, cannabis is not associated with serious side effects. Comparatively, the side effects of cannabis are mild and can often be addressed by switching products (those high in THC vs. CBD or other cannabinoids). For example, some cannabis products like THC, Delta-8, or CBN are dehydrating, and people who take them complain that their eyes and/or mouth may feel dry. Addressing dehydration is an easy fix—drink more water—and especially important for seniors, because it can lead to a loss of balance. Light-headedness is another manifestation of the drying effects cannabis can have. To counteract or prevent light-headedness, always use cannabis products when you can drink lots of water. What's more, be aware that consuming cannabis along with over-the-counter pharmaceuticals, such as antihistamines, as well as stimulants, heart medicines, antibiotics, and many others, might cause additional dryness, like dry mouth and dry skin.

Some of the most common side effects of cannabis include:

+ Agitation
+ Amplification of body sensations that cause feelings of anxiousness or paranoia
+ Amplification of emotions that cause feelings of anxiousness or paranoia
+ Confusion
+ Coughing (lung irritation from inhaling)
+ Dehydration
+ Dizziness
+ Drowsiness
+ Dry, bloodshot eyes
+ Dry mouth
+ Facial flushing
+ Illusions, delusions, and hallucinations (only at high doses)
+ Increased appetite
+ Increased blood pressure (although prolonged use may cause a decrease in blood pressure)
+ Increased heart rate (tachycardia)
+ Light-headedness
+ Nausea
+ Panic attacks
+ Reduced coordination
+ Restlessness
+ Short-term memory impairment
+ Time distortions
+ Tremors
+ Upset stomach

The most common complaint I hear from my patients is that their initial trial of a cannabis therapy made them feel too anxious. I can understand; trying anything new can be awkward. And when suffering is muted, we can be hyper-aware of our new state, which can initially feel uncomfortable. This anxiety surrounding new situations is what some people describe as *paranoia*, but to me it is nothing more than a manifestation of fear without understanding the true source.

Similarly, an upset stomach can sometimes occur as a reaction to an ingredient in the food or oil that is used in creating cannabis products. It can also be a reaction in the gut's nervous system—known as the enteric nervous system—to newness: a version of paranoia for your stomach. Over time, these anxiety-related side effects will dissipate as your system adjusts. Sometimes, just being aware that you may feel anxious is all it takes to keep paranoia at bay.

When you are using cannabis therapies, you can completely control every aspect of your experience, including side effects. For instance, you can change your dosage, your product, or the strengths of a particular formulation. What's more, the next time you try the same therapy, you will not likely have the same anxieties because you will have already experienced the new sensation.

I find that once people can pass through paranoia, everybody's happier with their therapy. I've helped dozens of people who came back to see me after a year or two years, telling me that they initially didn't like how cannabis made them feel, so they gave it up. However, nothing else was helping them, so they were willing to give it another try. The second time, I was able to help them with a slightly slower approach. One such patient, Brenda, decided to give cannabis gummies a try, after a shocking episode of sleepwalking associated with her prescription sleep medicine. Unfortunately, Brenda made the age-old mistake when desperate for an adequate night's rest—she took too many edibles. The unfortunate blend of frustration, disappointment, and too much THC thrust Brenda onto a sensory roller-coaster ride, which turned her off cannabis completely. Yet four years later, Brenda called me again. We worked out a dosage plan, and she now sets the clock to a ninety-minute countdown after eating an edible. Now she has plenty of time to finish up her day and get into bed and gets a refreshing, if not life-changing, consistent seven-hour rest per night.

There Are Plenty of Pleasant "Side Effects"

There's another category of cannabis "side effects" that are not only tolerable, but for many, enjoyable. For instance, many people who choose THC products may feel more relaxed and joyful while they are treating sleeplessness or pain. Depending on set and setting, product ingredients, and dosage, many of my patients experience greater sexual disinhibition, and an increase or decrease in sociability. Others have told me about enhanced productivity, creativity, and sensory perceptions, increasing their appreciation for art, music, and food.

I also know that there are people who purposefully isolate themselves from their feelings, who prevent themselves from experiencing any emotion. Cannabis has the ability to mute our defense mechanisms. If someone has walled off uncomfortable thoughts or emotions, cannabis can release those. You may at first find that tapping into a full range of emotions may be uncomfortable, yet the experience of accepting your emotions can be cathartic and therapeutic.

Control

Guided cannabis is nothing if not a flexible treatment option. It doesn't have a rigid schedule of administration that may be inconvenient. You can control how it will make you feel on any given day, choosing a product that is more relaxing or stimulating, or one that is short-acting as opposed to an extended-release variety. In short, you are the master of your own fate. Decisions about medicines can be folded in with nutrition and exercise choices, sleep habits, and matched with specific and ever-changing daily needs.

The reason that control is available is because of the inherent safety profile of cannabis. We don't have strong evidence that accidentally taking too much can hurt you in a permanent way. The same is not true for other pharmaceuticals, which is why they come with specific instructions on how much to take to avoid an ill effect. So not only can you choose what products are best for you, you can also fine-tune your search. You are limited in your ability to fine-tune the effects of Benadryl: you can take less than the maximum dose, but if you take more, you risk serious medical effects. But you can fine-tune the impact of different cannabis products in your body to an incredibly specific degree. This open-ended freedom can be abused, but I've found that the bulk of people who mistakenly take too much suffer temporary consequences of their extravagance, and learn not to repeat it.

With so much control in your own hands, your relationship with your health-care provider may change. The optimal relationship between you and your provider should take into account all of the pieces of your well-being, which includes sleep, nutrition, exercise, and now cannabis. Provided that they are educated about cannabis, they can partner with you to make good choices based on your current health profile. The process of obtaining medical access is different in each state, but it largely involves approval for a licensed provider to a patient who qualifies for state-approved health conditions. Once you have this access, dosing, frequency, and the specific regimen are rarely prescribed, which is why you are in control.

As such, we know ourselves best. We know what we are looking for. We know what we need on any given day. And we know that everything about our lives is adaptable. The way we feel physically or mentally can vary on a daily basis. The cannabis industry is growing in a wild, organic fashion where there are new products being launched all the time, and they all have subtle differences that may appeal to different situations for different people. Knowing yourself best means you can pick products that are most appropriate for you and take them on the schedule that works for you. You may find a product that is a better match for you on days where you feel more tired, and another when you need to feel less anxious.

Your cannabis treatment plan can change when your symptoms resolve or if the ever-changing circumstances of normal life interfere. Unlike medications that you have to be on regardless of symptoms, you will be able to simply stop using products when you feel better, and revisit them if symptoms return. Many patients have told me that they go on and off treatment as their needs change, and that level of adaptability is so different from traditional medications, like antidepressants or pain-management medications.

Adaptability

Cannabis can help us adapt to life and dial back the difficulty of living with discomfort. Because cannabis can redirect our focus while softening pain and amplifying signals of pleasure, it allows us to learn that pain does not have to be completely consuming of one's daily experience. This in and of itself can change your experience of illness. With more control of how you want to feel, you can decide how illness or pain is going to affect your life. You may find that you are less bothered by your discomfort, or that you choose not to pay attention to it. In this way, you can break the cycle of uninterrupted suffering so that you can get back to being your best self.

The reason why cannabis is so effective is that it has *adaptogenic* properties: it is a nontoxic plant that improves the body's ability to resist multiple forms of stress—including physical, chemical, and biological sources—by increasing its ability to adapt and survive.[4]

No matter how stressors are affecting the brain and body, adaptogens can help to bring us into balance. For example, if we are too anxious, they calm us down, and if we are depressed, they brighten up our mood. Like ashwagandha, lemon balm, and ginseng, which are true adaptogens that have been used in Chinese, Indian, and Western medicine to treat stress, cannabis can hack your perspective so that you can thrive, even in the presence of illness.

Lastly, the vast array of products available can help you continue to reap the benefits of cannabis. When a cannabinoid receptor interacts with the exact same cannabinoid molecule over and over again, the receptor actually *involutes*, or disappears into the host cell. This is what happens whenever we develop a tolerance to any type of medication: the receptors need more in order to continue to work. However, when there is a subtle variation in the army of cannabinoid products, their molecules will be different. By consuming different cannabis forms at varying times and volumes, you will get longer-lasting effects without creating a tolerance.

Ten Reasons to Get Past the Stigma and Feel Better

There's a pervasive misconception in our culture that cannabis is a substance that's bad for you. Even if you have been a recreational user in the past, we've all been conditioned to the institutional propaganda against cannabis: the way that American culture has systematically demonized people's use and the way that it is used in secrecy. It's time to overcome stigma and put aside the negative associations you may have heard about. If you've come this far, you are ready to try something new.

1. Cannabis isn't going to make you psychotic, but it will impact your brain. Everyone is born on a continuum with edges. Just as one can be on the border of too jumpy or too unmotivated, one can be living on the edge of madness. Cannabis consumed wisely with attention to terpenes and cannabinoids has helped countless people step back from the line of mental discomfort, smoothing out their edges to be able to achieve a consistent state. The vast majority of people who use cannabis regularly do so because they're enjoying the experience.

2. Cannabis isn't any more addictive than your morning cup of coffee or your afternoon run.

3. Cannabis is no more of a gateway drug than alcohol, and it doesn't have the hazardous side effects that come with drinking, such as headaches, nausea, blackouts, or the serious chronic conditions of liver disease, diabetes, obesity, and heart disease. Hangovers are rare and usually caused by inadequate hydration rather than the cannabis itself. Best of all, many of my patients who learn to medicate with cannabis rather than alcohol are surprised to feel happier, healthier, and better than ever.

4. Cannabis doesn't have the bungee rebound symptoms that prescription sleep aids have.

5. The costs of cannabis products are far lower than prescription drugs.

6. Cannabis can help undo the daily stressors of life by helping you unwind, set anxieties aside, and reset your brain and body with a good night's sleep.

7. Cannabis contains many of the same nutrients found in a well-rounded plant-based diet. It is a superfood like red wine, chocolate, blueberries, and other colorful fruits and vegetables.

8. You don't have to smoke cannabis to get its positive effects. In the next chapter, you will learn of the many options available for consumption.

9. Cannabis does not make you permanently "dopey," slow, or lazy. The myths around cannabis making people less dynamic or less flexible cognitively have not borne out through the test of time and study. In fact, the use of some products, such as CBD, in situations where someone needs

to remember will help enhance memory and increase productivity, focus, and attention.

10. Share your success! The more open you are to your use, the better you will feel. I've collected thousands of patient reports that connect better health outcomes with how open people are to communicating about their cannabis use with their immediate family, their friends, and even strangers. It's almost as if people derive more benefit when their community is aware of their use.

What's Next

Transitioning to cannabis therapies can be overwhelming. There are so many choices: what types of products to buy and where to buy them. The next chapter will help make these decisions easier.

CHAPTER 3

The Shopper's Guide to Cannabis Products

O ne of the wonderful aspects of cannabis medicine is that it offers a completely individualized approach to taking care of your health. The types of products that will work best for you can be completely different from what your partner or friends are using, even if you are treating the same conditions. The fact is: We are all very different. We have different genetics, we come in different sizes, we have different mindsets, likes and dislikes, and we live in different environments.

What's more, on different days or under different circumstances, we may have different preferences, or we may want to construct different types of relief. I am not the same person that I will be three hours from now, nor am I the same person I was a week ago, or three months ago. We are dramatically and constantly changing, on both a mental and physical level, down to our cells and ever-changing brain. And the world around us is constantly changing. Our environment is changing. The seasons are changing. The stress of daily life is changing. All of these factors affect how we interact with cannabis and how effective it is on any given day.

I know that this may seem like a very different approach to medicine. We've been taught that we should get the same result from the same dose of medication regardless of how we feel on a particular day, or what our environment is like. But the fact is, it's just not the case. It's a goal, but that goal is not always met, and perhaps it may never be met.

So how do we manage a protocol that is so affected by how we are changing if we are looking for reproducible and consistent results? The answer is to fully understand the vast array of products that are available, so that you have a complete arsenal to meet your daily, changing needs. That may mean different types of products as well as different strengths within the same type. Don't get hung up on a particular brand or name of a product: you really have to focus on the ingredient or series of ingredients. If it turns out that the product you are most comfortable with and is providing the most relief is a particular edible, you will want to also find other products with the same ingredients in case that edible is sold out. Even if you can get the same manufactured product that you liked last time, because it is based on a natural plant, there may likely be slight differences in its effectiveness because two plants are never identical. And, the product that worked for you last time, even if it's in an unopened package from the same manufacturer, may be less effective six months from now because the product is changing in small ways inside the packaging. However, don't dismay: the natural variability in product actually energizes our brain receptors for cannabinoids differently, which makes developing a tolerance less likely.

The ideal way to find the best set of products that work for your particular health concerns and unique conditions may require a little investigation. This chapter introduces all of the different products that are typically available. You may need to test-drive several types to see which works for you, and then rank your choices so that you have a backup plan in case the one you want is not available. You may also want to purchase in bulk if you find something that is particularly helpful.

Quick Product Overview

There are many ways to use and consume cannabis, and each of them has different properties and useful functions:

+ Balms
+ Bath products (bath bombs, salts)

+ Capsules (filled with oil concentrates or tinctures)
+ Combustion products (joint, bowl, chillum)
+ Dissolving tablets/strips
+ Edibles
+ Eye drops
+ Flower (nugget, seeds, sticks, leaves, roots, or kief)
+ Infusion products (carbonated and still beverages, drink drops)
+ Lotions
+ Nebulizers
+ Nose drops
+ Oral spray
+ Patches
+ Salves
+ Suppositories
+ Teas
+ Tinctures
+ Topicals
+ Vaporizer: concentrate
+ Vaporizer: flower
+ Wax: full-spectrum and its derivatives (full extract cannabis oil [FECO], Rick Simpson Oil [RSO], hash, rosin, live sugar)
+ Wax: isolated derivatives in many forms (shatter, budder, powder, crystals)
+ Wine

At caplancannabis.com, you will find a gallery of images, diagrams, and more information about these products.

Edibles

Edibles as a category includes all foods, snacks, and beverages that have been infused with cannabinoids. The variety is as wide as your imagination: There are chocolates, mints, candies, honey sticks, lozenges, chewing gum, and gummies.

You can buy cannabis pizzas, cookies, peanut butter, and hazelnut spread. There are teas, wines, and carbonated drinks. There are "drops" or "squeeze" products available, which offer you an option to medicate whatever beverage you already have at home. What's more, new products are coming to the marketplace regularly.

The soft tissues of the mouth and throat readily and rapidly absorb cannabinoid molecules. Tissues under the tongue, along the cheeks, and along the lining of the throat have dense highways of blood vessels that provide a convenient on-ramp to absorb cannabinoids. The digestive process then absorbs the cannabinoids from edibles relatively slowly, unless they are made with a high oil content, which can be absorbed more rapidly and can have a faster onset of effects. A process called *nanotechnology emulsification*, in which cannabinoids become water soluble, can further increase the absorption of cannabis into the body: it is a technology that allows cannabis to be diluted evenly within a drink, and aids its ability to cross water barriers inside the body more easily.

Many users are drawn to edibles as the doses are easier to control, they are more discreet than vaping, and there is no risk of airway irritation. Edibles differ from inhalation and tinctures that are dissolved under the tongue because, rather than have the cannabinoids enter directly into the bloodstream, the cannabinoids are first processed, or metabolized, in the digestive system. By first metabolizing the cannabinoids, users are actually circulating a product formed from the cannabinoids, known as *metabolites*. The metabolic process is part of the reason edibles take longer to affect users. *Metabolites* is a term that describes an end or intermediate product of metabolism and is not specific to cannabis. The metabolites act on the endocannabinoid system differently than other products and are frequently more potent that the original cannabinoid.

The effects from edibles tend to last a long time, even at low dosages. A typical starting dose is 5 milligrams (mg) of a 1:1 ratio of CBD:THC edible candy. This could be individually wrapped portions or a small square of a 100 mg chocolate bar (one can be divided into twenty small pieces). This balance of THC/CBD is generally felt to be pleasant without being too powerful: it can be taken during any part of the day.

If you want to avoid sugar, especially in candy products, look for edibles that are sugar-free. The sugar component of edibles will be absorbed more rapidly than the cannabinoids: you will feel the ebb and flow of energy changes due to the sugar content in addition to the cannabinoid effect.

General Rules for Edibles

1. The effects of edibles may begin 30–120 minutes after consumption, depending on your hydration level and how recently you ate a large meal. Set a timer for one hour from when you first swallow it. The effects of edibles tend to begin when the timer goes off, unless you have taken the edible following a large meal. Conversely, eating an edible on an empty stomach can decrease the time of onset and increase the potency of effects.

2. Gummies and sugar-based candies typically last four to seven hours.

3. Choosing edible cannabis products that are high in natural fats (butter, fat, oils) often extends their duration of effects. Chocolate-based products often have a longer-lasting effect than gummies because of their higher dietary fat/oil content.

4. To avoid one edible amplifying the effects of another, limit yourself to one edible within a two-hour period.

5. Begin with low dosages (2–5 mg) of THC and/or products that contain more CBD than THC.

6. No effect at all may be preferable to an uncomfortable result. If an effect is small and pleasant, continue using the same dosage, as needed. If no effect occurs, increase your dosage by 2 mg per day, until you have realized the desired effect.

7. If you achieve a positive effect, but it is not reproducible over time, increase the dosage incrementally.

Marketing Terms You Need to Know

The cannabis marketplace has adopted a number of terms that refer to the level of energy you may feel when taking products. These terms are used to describe both THC and CBD products, and are far more accurate than simply "sativa or indica" that are often used with THC products, or merely a named cannabis strain:

+ Indica or calming/sedating/quieting/nighttime
+ Hybrid/neutral or day-or-night energy
+ Sativa or energizing/activating/stimulating

Topicals

Topicals have penetrative effects that allow them to function optimally when applied to the superficial layers of skin. Internal topicals that can penetrate mucus membranes include suppositories, eye drops, and nose drops.

Topical Options

DISPENSARY TOPICALS	CBD/ONLINE TOPICALS
+ Dispensaries typically carry THC options, but sometimes carry 1:1 THC:CBD varieties. + There are a variety of thickness options. The thicker the better. The occlusive nature of thicker balms usually means they have more obstructive power, which prevents evaporation and propels more effective penetration into the skin. + Look for a minimum of 400 mg of active cannabinoids per 4–6 ounces of product.	+ Look for multiple aromatic ingredients (not just pure CBD, but products that also include lavender, lemon, mint), which means that they have added terpenes. + Ideally, look for about 400 mg of active cannabinoids in a 10-ounce product.

The most effective topicals add terpenes to their formulations, either directly from cannabis plants or from other plants. These terpenes may have unique and interesting smells as well as other medicinal qualities, and many also affect the depth and speed with which the cannabis can diffuse into body tissues. Effective topicals can be found both online and in dispensaries, although they may have different properties.

General Rules for Topicals:

1. The effects of topicals may begin within one to two minutes of application, and often last one to two hours.

2. There is no known maximum dose, so you can feel confident to reapply topicals liberally and as often as necessary without concern for adverse reactions. We don't see tolerance effects either, so similar doses seem to be effective indefinitely.

3. When topicals work well (i.e., when they penetrate effectively, in terms of depth and speed), both CBD and THC products seem to have similar effects. The ratio of CBD:THC doesn't seem to relate to its effectiveness. As long as the molecule finds a receptor to bind to, they will have the same response.

4. THC topicals are *not* associated with euphoria. Even when topicals are used on the face or neck, which are areas close to the brain, they only contain a small percentage of cannabinoids, and by the time they reach the brain, they've already survived several passes through the bloodstream, including some degradation processes.

5. Topicals can be used in combination with other methods of cannabis and with other topical medicines.

6. Topicals with a high oil-to-water ratio may feel greasy or leave marks on clothing. Applying a Band-Aid or other covering on top of topicals will keep your clothes clean and help increase the durability of its effects.

Tinctures

Alcohol- or oil-based solutions of THC and/or CBD are packaged in a liquid vial with a medicine dropper. They offer a relatively dilute concentration of cannabinoids along with the producer's choice of additives, which can include terpenes and flavonoids or botanicals, flavors, or colors. Some products add melatonin as a sleep aid, or caffeine as a stimulant, or other commonly used supplement ingredients to amplify their effects with cannabinoids.

When solutions are mixed with an oil-based solvent, the technical term is *infusion*; when they are mixed with alcohol, it is referred to as a *tincture*. For the sake of simplicity, we, and the larger cannabis marketplace, refers to both as *tinctures*.

Tinctures are a great option if you want to titrate a specific dose to take regularly. You can easily control the number of drops taken, and when you use a medicine dropper, the drops are about the same size. If today's dose isn't optimal, adding one or two drops the following session (after at least three to four hours) is a reasonable way to advance to a more successful dosage.

Read labels carefully: the concentration of active ingredients can be diluted. To ensure that you are getting the dosage you want, purchase a calibrated dropper from your local drugstore so that you have a measuring tool to understand where your comfort zone is, and your dose can be replicated. With standard droppers, one dropperful is roughly 1 millileter (mL) of liquid. There are approximately 20–25 drops per 1 mL of liquid. Check the label of the tincture bottle to see how many milligrams of active ingredients are in each drop or dropperful. Compare this information to the chart on page 65 to determine your starting point.

Tinctures made with an oil base will tend to last longer in the system than alcohol-based varieties. When taken by mouth, alcohol tinctures are known to have a bite or sting to them, but they often work more rapidly than their oil counterparts. However, the vast majority of tinctures sold in the marketplace are oil-based. Both oil and alcohol tinctures can be easily made at home, and the instructions are in the following chapter.

Tinctures can also be ingested as capsules, placed into appropriate pH-balanced suppositories, or inhaled through nebulization. A nebulizer is a mechanical tool used to breathe in medication via tubing, avoiding the irritation of smoke and the heat of vaporized products. Only cannabis tinctures made with whole grain alcohol can be used in nebulizer formulations; the alcohol portion evaporates before it would be inhaled into the body.

Tincture Options

OIL-BASED TINCTURES (INFUSIONS)	ALCOHOL-BASED TINCTURES
+ May work through the skin if applied topically	+ May work through the skin if applied topically
+ Application under the tongue works faster than swallowed	+ May work more quickly under the tongue than oil-based
+ May be added to drinks and foods	+ Can be used inside room humidifiers or diffusers, as well as personal nebulizers
	+ Small amounts are not associated with alcohol intoxication

General Rules for Tinctures

1. Shake the tincture bottle well to ensure an even distribution of ingredients. Measure out your starting dose.

2. Place drops under the tongue and hold for ninety seconds before swallowing. Or, hold the dropper over a spoon and gently squeeze out the number of drops you want. Then swallow with a glass of water.

3. The effects of tinctures may begin in thirty to sixty minutes, and often last for four to five hours.

4. Use caution when taking tinctures at the same time as other cannabis products. Depending on whether or not the body is already exposed to cannabinoids from inhalation or an edible, even a few drops of tincture can build on an otherwise satisfactory experience of cannabis. In some cases, this gentle augmentation can prolong beneficial effects, but in others, the extra dose of tincture cannabinoids can become nauseating, sedating, or induce feelings of anxiety or paranoia.

Inhalation Options: Flower and Flower Derivatives

The purest form of cannabis that you can buy is the flower, pulled right off the plant. While the entire cannabis plant produces cannabinoids, including the sticks, leaves, and roots, none are quite as potent and concentrated in cannabinoids as the flower portion, called a *cola* when it is dried. The most medicinal part of the flower is called *kief*, the dried trichomes containing THC, CBD, terpenes, and flavonoids. Smoked flower using a joint, bowl, bong, chillum, and so on aerosolizes the kief and uses the other leafy plant parts as a wick to continuously heat various sections of the flower.

There are people who have smoked in the past and continue to love smoking because of the instantaneity of its effects. Smoking involves heating cannabis to very high temperatures, which yields a fast reaction time and a larger release of cannabinoids: the hotter the compound that's coming in, the more intense the effect is likely to be, as cannabinoids can vault into the bloodstream directly and efficiently. Yet exposing body tissues, such as the mouth and throat, to extreme heat accompanies increased blood flow to the exposed surfaces, which is why you may feel discomfort in the back of your throat, or cough, when you smoke.

What's more, smoking is probably the most obviously harmful method of consuming cannabinoids over the long term, which is why I don't recommend it, particularly for the uninitiated. Smoking brings harmful compounds into the body, including ash, carbon monoxide, and tar, the same toxins that are also found in tobacco cigarettes. Tar is sticky and can affix to your teeth or lung tissue, as well as to your furniture, rugs, and clothing, often leaving lasting odors and sediment.

However, I do understand that medicine is often a risk-benefit analysis. And there are some people for whom no other cannabis product seems to work quite as well as smoking. It may be as simple as embracing the familiarity: old habits die hard, and exploring new methods can be daunting. I can't stress enough the importance of at least trying other options. Even some of my long-time smokers find real benefits in avoiding even subtle lung changes, especially as they get older.

You also need to consider cost as a factor. From a financial point of view, smoking flower directly is the most wasteful option. It's not that flower is expensive, but the cost per experience equation does not work in smoking's favor. For example, one gram of cannabis flower, the typical size of a joint, might last for two sessions. In contrast, taking one-third of a gram and putting it into a vaporizer that can be set with temperature precision, could yield three sessions, so that one gram could last a full nine sessions. What's more, when you smoke flower, you cannot reuse the ash. After you vaporize flower, on the other hand, the residue can be used to create a tincture, because many of the cannabinoids are still available even after it's been vaped. Lastly, vaping temperatures are usually about one-tenth of the temperatures reached by smoking, and they are still effective at releasing nearly the full amount of cannabinoids.

Vaping

Vaping is shorthand for consuming aerosolized cannabinoids via a vaporizer. Individual cannabinoids, when heated to precise boiling-point temperatures, can be aerosolized into the lungs using a vaporizer. There are various types of vaporizers: some heat the cannabis with direct contact, while others act indirectly. A convection vaporization, for example, warms cannabis with a device that includes a fan underneath the heating system. The fan blows hot air through cannabinoid concentrate or flower into a conduit, which can then be inhaled. Conduction vaporization puts direct contact between the product and a heat source. Cannabis vapor pens (and their nicotine-based counterparts) operate using this principle: they use a small hot plate to vaporize concentrate, which then travels through a tiny mouthpiece. If this is your preferred method, invest in a high-quality vapor pen: the inexpensive options are often made cheaply and can emit toxic metal particles into your lungs. Dispensaries offer the purest regulated products that will not include additives that may be dangerous when inhaled. Although the degree to which dispensaries regulate the purity of their products varies, all regulated stores provide tested vaping products that are safe from such toxins.

Vaping is much safer than smoking. The problems you may have heard of pertaining to vapor cartridges back in 2019 have been resolved. Those issues involved homemade products and were never associated with cannabinoid cartridges that were professionally produced. However, most of us grew up learning that anything we inhale that isn't air—particularly "smoke"—was akin to swallowing air pollution. In fact, vaporized cannabis products are generally well tolerated and are not associated with the toxins or the intense heat of smoking. It's always a risk-benefit equation: you may be giving up instant results for a healthier solution. So just like everything else about this cannabis journey, you will have to pick the product that best suits your needs.

Cannabis Concentrates/Distillates

Besides flower, you can also purchase different blends of cannabis concentrates. These come as a wax or other oily substances, all derived from kief. Concentrates and distillates are a highly purified form of cannabis and can be very potent. They are sold by weight at dispensaries, or you can make your own.

There are many ways to heat the waxy forms: by direct or indirect heat sources, as part of combustion, or some combination. Or you can expose cannabis concentrate to a heat source, and inhale the vapor that results. For example, you could use a device called a dab rig: this is a metal nail that heats up to red-hot temperatures. You place a small amount of concentrate on top (called a dab), then wait about a half minute for the nail to cool to its original color, which signifies that the temperature of the dab is appropriate for building a puff of cannabis. On contact, the heat from the nail instantly vaporizes the concentrate into a cloud of particles that can then be inhaled.

Vaping Cannabis and Cannabis Concentrate Options

The three types of vaporizer products—flower, flower + concentrate, and concentrate alone—range in potency. Specific products are geared to specific categories. For example, there are certain vape pens that only support concentrates, and others that are made for flower or flower/concentrate. Make sure your product matches your vehicle of use.

FLOWER	FLOWER + CONCENTRATE	PURE CONCENTRATES
Least potent	*Variable potency (adjustable)*	*High potency*
+ Heat in a vaporizer at specific temperatures	+ Used with a vaporizer	+ Fast-acting, potent, minimal puffs required (1 puff + 2 minutes wait before next puff)
+ Effect is slow to begin, and ramps up gently with progressive inhalations	+ Sprinkle a dusting of kief onto flower for a mild increase in potency	+ Increase frequency and/or size of inhalations
+ Inhale with frequent or continuous pulls	+ Add a thin strand of wax or shatter to flower for additional potency	+ Available as both THC and CBD-only concentrates
	+ Added concentrate may amplify the overall effects of the mixture	

General Rules for Vaporization

1. The onset of effects begins more slowly with vaporized flower than with concentrates, and much faster than edibles. Vaping can yield results within seconds and last anywhere from one to three hours.
2. A vape concentrate may require as little as one puff to achieve goal effects, so it is easy to vaporize too much at once. Waiting two minutes between puffs can help with recognition and regulation of effects.
3. Vaporized cannabis can be inhaled multiple times over the course of an hour and stopped once a desired effect is achieved. In order to sustain that level of efficacy, you may need to continue vaping. This is one option for following a microdosing strategy (see page 68).

4. Choose the inhalation technique you are most comfortable with, and then stick to that process as much as possible so that you can achieve a consistent result. Consider the type of breathing (deep diaphragmatic breathing or shallow mouth breaths), the shape of your lips and mouth to create a vacuum, the speed of your inhalations, and whether you're holding the vapor in or not.

5. For someone who's never vaped, first try a temperature-controlled vaporizer that heats only flower. Alternate breaths with and without cannabis: breathe a full, deep breath in with cannabis vapor coming into the lungs, and then take a couple breaths that are without cannabis. Repeat until you feel the desired effect; then stop and wait ten minutes to see if the effects match your expectation.

6. Varying the ratios and individual amounts of CBD, THC, and terpene content drastically alters the effects of any inhaled product.

Prescription Medications

Your healthcare provider can prescribe cannabis pharmaceutical formulations to treat very specific illnesses and conditions. As with most medications, any of these can be prescribed for off-label use.

+ **Dronabinol (Marinol):** a capsule or a solution used to treat AIDS-related anorexia, nausea, and vomiting, including during chemotherapy
+ **Sativex:** an oral mucosal spray that is 1:1 THC:CBD used to treat pain in advanced cancer patients and multiple sclerosis (currently available outside the US)
+ **Epidiolex:** a pure CBD formulation used to treat seizures associated with Dravet syndrome and Lennox-Gastaut syndrome

Avoiding Ineffective Products

CBD products are effective, yet they have a bad reputation because they are so ubiquitous: you can buy them on the internet, at big retailers like Whole Foods, or at independent CBD stores that might have just popped up in your local mall or neighborhood. And because these products are not sold in pharmacies or dispensaries, which are regulated institutions, you are trusting that the safeguards of modern capitalism will ensure that the CBD products contain what they advertise. So how do you make sure that you are getting what you paid for?

The answer is simple: review the labels and sellers carefully, and look for products that have been tested by independent third-party laboratories. These labs exist throughout the world, and even the smallest manufacturers and at-home producers, can have their products rigorously tested for purity and safety. Third-party verifiers use a safety standard and ingredients checklist referred to as a *certificate of analysis* (COA). You can see if a product has a recent COA by checking out its website, or by inquiring directly with the manufacturer.

A second issue that affects CBD potency is how these mass-produced products are stored. For instance, if an edible product is left in the sun, different components that react to heat or humidity may melt or mutate, and its therapeutic effects can change. Similarly, depending upon the mixture of ingredients combined with the cannabinoids—the sugar, oil, fruit essence, or other nutraceutical content—the end product may have a different physiological impact. Just as all medicines have a shelf life, both cannabinoids and the ingredients mixed with them can deteriorate over time, and their efficacy changes. Knowing how fresh a product is, in addition to precisely what went into the product, is critical to understanding one's experience and facilitating reproducible results.

If you are unhappy with a product, investigate before you toss it away. There are many ways to adjust an unsatisfying cannabinoid product to make it work to your advantage. For instance, if you want to get a better night's sleep, try CBD edibles. If you start with the lowest dose and take it for a week and nothing happens, how do you know whether to increase the dose or switch to a different product?

Most companies that are producing CBD are basically producing versions of the same products with different strengths or additives. You are buying a specific concentration of CBD floating in an oil with variations in flavors and other active ingredients. Some companies play around with each of these components, including the amount of CBD or the amount of oil, and occasionally, the producers may add a different oil to see if that works better. By altering the amount of

CBD per total amount consumed, or by adjusting the timing when you take it, it is possible to discover your sweet spot for CBD-improved sleep with the product you already have.

Dosing: Where Should I Start?

When it comes to cannabis, there are no hard and fast "prescriptions" in the traditional medical model of form, frequency, and dose. Dispensaries and other types of retailers aren't pharmacies that are following instructions from healthcare providers, and outside of Germany, Uruguay, and select other countries, pharmacies themselves only provide prescription (pharmaceutical) cannabis. Clinicians can't tell the marketplace what plants to grow, nor which products they should stock or supply. What's more, the consistency of products to purchase depends more on the manufacturer's own revenue strategies than what may provide the most medical benefit to any specific patient.

As mentioned earlier in the chapter, these variables may seem like a liability, but to my mind, they provide an opportunity to achieve control with the products that work for you, as long as you have self-awareness about what product success looks like for you, and an understanding of the marketplace and the range of products sold. The rest of this chapter will help you reach a scientifically informed decision so that you can make the right purchases and provide effective self-care.

The aim for optimizing your dosage is to create an experience that is not overwhelming or overly intense: attaining subtle improvements that will not interrupt your usual daily experience and offer long-standing improvement. From there you can further fine-tune your dosing for maximal relief. The individual chapters in part II will make targeted recommendations for specific illnesses and conditions; the information here is merely a starting point.

The following chart provides information on typical THC dosages in products that are available at dispensaries and retail stores. Details on specific products and their consumption have been listed in the previous pages. When purchasing, look for a packaged product that matches the exact dose you require. However, there may be times when what you need is not available; you can purchase larger dose items and separate them into smaller dosages.

It's important to remember how different each product is from others in the same category. Please read labels carefully and note dosage information, which is more valuable and relevant to you than "serving size." If you are not consuming the entire product in one sitting, you may want to record the dosage information for later use.

The strength of THC products can be modified if they include CBD or other terpenes. For instance, the presence of CBD and/or some terpenes in higher dosage products may soften the cognitive effects, but may increase the cognitive impacts of lower dosages.

Comparing Typical THC Dosages

DOSE	DOSE STRENGTH	EFFECT EXPECTATIONS
1 mg	Microdose	Minimal impact. Very subtle effect on cognition, if felt at all. Good choice for repeated use over the course of a day. Microdosing avoids intense sensations.
2.5 mg	Low	Small impact. For new consumers, this is a typical starting dose. Effects are noticeable but not overwhelming, unless you have previously been sensitive to other medicines. Small impact on cognition.
3–5 mg	Low–med	Small impact. New consumers may feel noticeable but not overwhelming effects, including euphoria and changes in perception and coordination. Experienced users often choose 5 mg as a beginning dose.
7.5 mg	Med	Low–moderate impact. Effects can be strong and potentially overwhelming. Should be taken with a full glass of water. Experienced users are rarely overwhelmed at this level.

DOSE	DOSE STRENGTH	EFFECT EXPECTATIONS
10 mg	Med	Moderate impact. New consumers will feel cognitive effects. Should be taken with a full glass of water. Experienced users may be able to tolerate without issues.
15–25 mg	Med–high	Distinct impact. New and experienced users will be cognitively affected.
50 mg	High	Powerful impact. May stay in the system for a full day. New and experienced consumers will feel strongly affected. Psychological and physical benefits will be robust and powerful, but typical side effects may be likely for new consumers. Fifty mg or more of pure CBD may elicit a noticeable state of relaxation.
100 mg +	Macrodose	Intensely intoxicating. Will stay in the system for at least 1 day. New and experienced consumers will feel strongly affected. Psychological and physical benefits will be robust and extremely powerful, but side effects are likely to occur for new consumers.

Cannabis Journaling Guidelines

If you'd like to formalize your assessments of the subtle differences in the experiences you will have with a range of products, record your notes in a journal or on a digital platform such as the EO Care app. Journaling cannabis use will help you track the experience, the benefits of different methods, and any associated environmental factors.

At the end of each day, track the following aspects of your routine:

Therapy goals: Identify your goals of treatment, both short term and long term. Your goals may change over time as certain conditions resolve or other concerns arise. You may find that when you successfully address certain health issues, like poor sleep, you will notice other aspects of your health improving, such as better attention or reduced pain.

Cannabis product: Record the name, date of purchase, place of purchase, and lot number of each product. Include any products you created at home. Laboratory testing results will inform you on subtle changes in products, such as terpenes, so that you can better understand what works best for you. For each product, record the ingredients, including percentage of:

+ THC
+ Delta-8-THC
+ CBD
+ CBN
+ CBC
+ CBGA
+ CBDV
+ THCA
+ THCV
+ Terpene
+ Flavonoids

Cannabis dosage/timing: Record how much you took, how often, and any other information relevant to administration (with food, with water, after exercise, how many hours before bedtime, etc.).

Other medications/supplements/lifestyle changes: Record medicines and supplements taken on the same day (timing, dosage, etc.) as your cannabis use to observe any relationships. Tracking daily exercise, food choices, and sleep schedule along with cannabis use will illustrate how well these systems work together.

> **Effect/symptom relief:** Record overall thoughts and experience, including how you respond to the four factors: peacefulness, comfort, control, and adaptability. When you can see that your health is improving over time, it's easier to stick with the program and share your results. Or, after a few weeks, if you notice that a particular product isn't working, you will have a record of what you've tried already as you look to find a better match for your needs.

Dosing Techniques: Macrodosing versus Microdosing

There are two dosing strategies that you can experiment with, regardless of what form of cannabis you are trying. They are related to size and frequency: how many times you are ingesting a product, and at what dosage.

The first strategy is referred to as *macrodosing*, which means taking a larger amount to achieve a single, robust therapeutic effect. Macrodosing is a more effective strategy when you are looking for an immediate effect, especially for sleep or pain relief. It's like taking a handful of mints at one time: you'll have really fresh breath for an hour. However, you may find that macrodosing THC is a bit overwhelming at first, and it will take your body longer to process out. The standout advantage of macrodosing is to pack a bigger punch aimed at an immediate effect.

Microdosing refers to the practice of consuming small amounts of cannabis in order to maximize the benefits while avoiding psychoactive effects that hinder everyday tasks. Microdosing is especially popular among those suffering from depression, anxiety, stress, and pain as it is particularly helpful when attempting to focus or fall asleep.

Just as with macrodosing, you can microdose with edibles, topicals, or inhalants. In this method, the cannabinoid levels slowly build throughout the day. By maintaining low dosages, precision dosing is easier to achieve, because you reach steady states more predictably than if you took a big dose. It's more like eating one mint every hour to have consistent fresh breath. Microdosing also minimizes the

psychological effects of THC products because you don't achieve sufficient receptor activation to feel overburdening euphoric effects.

There is no definite dosage chart to follow for microdosing cannabis due to the
various chemical compositions and the way you might process those chemicals at
different rates compared to someone else. It is commonly recommended that when
attempting to microdose, start with 2.5 mg, working up to 10 mg if necessary.
Wait at least an hour before taking the next dose.

Figure 3.1: What Microdosing Looks Like

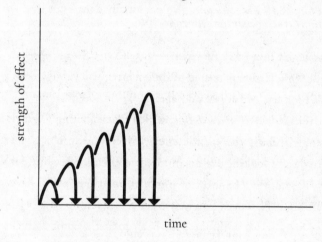

Figure 3.2: What Macrodosing Looks Like

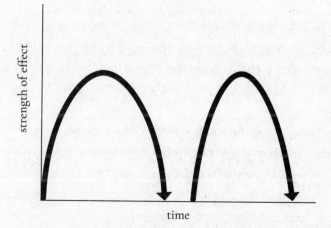

How Much Cannabis Is Too Much?

Consuming lots of large doses of cannabis can actually diminish the consistency of the medical benefits it provides. The reason is that too much cannabis in your system overpowers the ability of cannabinoid receptors to transmit a consistent, therapeutic action, and eventually, you will quickly develop a tolerance for the treatment. Developing a tolerance is like the experience of getting used to taking hot showers. The more often you are exposed to hot water, the less satisfying warm showers might be. Over time, you are going to have to crank up the hot water closer to a potentially dangerous level in order to feel satisfied.

Maintaining a low tolerance for cannabinoids improves the medical effects, and when you decrease the amount consumed, you also make your treatment more affordable. If you notice yourself consuming a large amount of product and not gaining the same benefit you are used to, abstain from use for forty-eight hours and then slowly reintroduce the product.

While tolerance to cannabis can build, the risk of a dependency seems to threaten the wallet more than the body. You know you have reached an excessive use of cannabis when:

+ The cost of maintaining your use becomes prohibitive.
+ The people around you comment on your cannabis use with concern.
+ You are continuing to use cannabis despite physical or psychological problems that didn't exist before cannabis use. These could be repeated or severe bouts of vomiting, irritability, headache, body ache, or lethargy despite trials with a variety of products.
+ You have severe withdrawal symptoms. Withdrawal symptoms are normal, but severe withdrawal symptoms that don't abate with a small amount of cannabis are a sign that you are using too much. Watch for irritability, headache, body ache, fever, chills, or lethargy.
+ You are giving up or reducing other activities in favor of cannabis.
+ You are taking cannabis in high-risk situations that show a lapse of good judgment: driving, operating machinery, and so on.

> - ✦ You are consistently taking more cannabis than you know you need to resolve your health problem.
> - ✦ You have difficulty controlling or cutting down your cannabis use.
> - ✦ You have problems at work, school, and home as a result of cannabis use.
>
> If you find that you are overusing, seek medical advice. In the very short term, a hot shower may help alleviate symptoms, especially if you are vomiting.

The Four Decisions

When choosing the optimal dosage, there are four core decisions to consider.

Choice #1: How Long Does It Take to Begin to Work?

- ✦ Quick acting: topicals, vaping   5–10 minutes
- ✦ Medium acting: patches, tinctures, gummies, candy   15–40 minutes
- ✦ Slow acting: suppositories, edibles, oil, capsules   30–120 minutes

Certain ailments are better served with specific products that are either fast or slow release. For example, people who experience sharp and sudden attacks of anxiety may find that having a cannabis product with effects that take hold in mere seconds is invaluable. On the other hand, there are many cannabinoid-based therapies that don't offer instant gratification, but instead support a steady foundation of relief to get one through an entire day.

A second issue around timing is whether you want your treatment protocol to be daytime appropriate or nighttime appropriate. For the majority of people, cannabis is consumed after work, between 5 and 9 PM at night, in a ritual process of unwinding and disentangling from the day's events, in the safety of one's home when you won't be driving, operating machinery, or making important decisions. However, as the cannabis industry has matured, options for lower-dosed products have become more popular, and more people are considering how a morning use of cannabinoids may help them become more productive or successful during the daytime, while avoiding distracting intoxication.

Choice #2: How Long Do the Effects Last?

Different product formulations as well as methods of consumption are either purposefully fast acting or have a delayed action.

- ✦ Vaping, tinctures, gummies, candy   45 minutes–4 hours
- ✦ Topicals, edibles, oil, capsules   4–8 hours
- ✦ Suppositories, patches   1–2 days

Cannabis has a short-term time window, which means that it has an immediate effect while you are consuming it. Additionally, remnants of it also remain in your bloodstream because it is stored in the fat cells of the body, and a little bit is released over time. As two to three weeks roll by, one's fat cells become saturated with consistent use—enough that they're going to be releasing therapeutic cannabis, even if you're not taking it immediately. In this way, yesterday's dose will add to today's in a small increment, and similarly add to tomorrow's. I've noticed that after about a week of taking cannabis regularly, my patients who use it for pain or sleep don't need to take it every day, because there's enough in their system to provide the relief they are looking for.

Imagine the ideal body buildup of cannabis to be like fueling a warm fire. At a consistent rate of fuel, the fire can be soothing and comfortable. Add too much fuel, and discomfort can come quickly and aggressively. There is a sweet spot: if you are consuming less than four days a week, you won't develop a meaningful tolerance; I have thousands of patients who are consuming cannabis a few days a week, and are on the same dose they've been on for years.

To increase a desired effect:

- ✦ After beginning with a small dose, advance slowly toward a minimum effective dose.
- ✦ Advance low dosages either by increasing amount (2 mg > 4 mg > 5 mg > 10 mg) or increasing the frequency (once daily > twice > three times daily).

Choice #3: Do You Want to Be High or Not High?

For some people, the euphoric effect that accompanies THC products is delightful and interesting, and they can't get enough of it. For other people, it is awkward, uncomfortable, and unsettling. My advice is to keep an open mind. If you've had a bad experience with smoking cannabis in the past, that doesn't mean you can't handle THC products and should avoid them. In reality, you probably were exposed to too much THC at one time. It's very common for people who take too much THC to feel out of sorts, so if you want to try THC products, erring on the side of underdosing will be more comfortable at first, yet possibly less effective and less pleasurable. Over time, you may become accustomed to THC naturally, and higher doses will be both better tolerated and more effective.

Luckily, you can now choose the degree to which your thought patterns are affected. Generally speaking, THC can offer a welcome washing away of recurring stress or sad thoughts, yet for some, this change in mindset can be off-putting, and clearheaded relaxation of the body is preferable. My clinical approach is almost always cautious. I would rather someone experience no relief at all, at first, than anything that makes them uncomfortable, pessimistic, or derails them. That means I often recommend to start with low doses, using THC-containing products at a bare minimum, at least for first-time users, because there's little risk of unsettling mind alteration. If you are just starting out and hoping to discover choices for lasting relief, look toward high-CBD, low-THC products.

CBD products work more powerfully on the body and are used to relax muscle tissues and bring about an overall level of calm. THC products are less effective on the body but are better for altering mental health issues because they affect the brain in a more direct, influential way. For those who have had experience with THC, a mixture of CBD and THC can feel dramatically less satisfying than pure THC. The appeal of THC is that you will find relief for your symptoms, and at the same time, will have an all-encompassing experience of joy. Lastly, THC is often associated with appetite stimulation and is used to treat a loss of appetite, while CBD is typically associated with the opposite effect, reducing appetite and/or reversing the appetite-stimulating effects of THC.

CBD is also used as an antidote for the euphoric aspects of THC. When they are mixed, the dominating properties of the individual molecules overlap, which sometimes cancels out their primary effects. CBD will help counteract the cognitive/psychotropic effects of THC when taken together. In case of unpleasant effects from cannabis, CBD may reverse (or help prevent) an uncomfortable experience. For some people exploring cannabis, time is of the essence, and trialing slowly may not be the desired path forward. Rather than starting with small doses of cannabinoids, you could try a product with both CBD and THC, so that less THC will bind into receptors, and the CBD acts to protect from the uncomfortable feelings associated with THC. Yet for some people, the two types of cannabinoid molecules appear to serve a synergistic relationship rather than a competitive one, and their experience is not subdued by CBD, but rather augmented by it.

There is literature that points to positive effects at a 20:1 ratio (20 CBD to 1 THC),[1] and I have found that it is a good ratio for the uninitiated. Oftentimes the effectiveness of the enhanced CBD is sufficient to achieve effective relief for most physical ailments, and it easily avoids altering mental status for those who are particularly worried about the effects of THC. Another benefit is that this type of product can be used at any time, at work or home. The downside is that the psychological relaxation effects of THC are absent, and for those who would benefit from more psychological relief, CBD-dominant choices don't seem to do quite as well.

Finally, don't be surprised if you change your preferred type of product. In my experience, people don't usually stay fixed to the camp in which they start. I've had patients who have consumed THC for years and love the euphoric feeling, yet once they discover that CBD products are effective without the intoxication, they end up enjoying a mix of CBD and THC. Conversely, people who are intimidated by THC tend to open up to the idea of it and find it quite ameliorating.

To minimize euphoric effects:

+ Look for products containing a higher ratio of CBD, CBG, THCA, CBDA, CBCA, or CBC, or supplement other regimens with high doses of these.
+ Products with CBD ratios greater than 3:1 (CBD to THC) are less likely to provide euphoric results.

+ The greater the ratio of CBD to THC (4:1, 6:1, 20:1), the less intoxicating.
+ Citrus fruits, black pepper, caffeine, water, sleep, exercise, and time also help cancel the intoxicating effects. The sooner you can try these antidotes in relation to the timing of the THC dosage, the more effective they are.

Choice #4: What Is Your Energy Goal?

+ Sativa: invigorating, energizing, activating
+ Hybrid: neutral energy, delicately elevating, generally pleasing
+ Indica: calming, relaxing, sedating

The individual compounds within the various types of cannabis plants include a massive spectrum of aromatic and sensory-stimulating molecules that have direct effects on human receptors. To convey the meaning and generalizable effects of this complicated chemistry, the terms *sativa* and *indica* are used to convey some of the dominant effects those molecules will have. In the marketplace, you'll find a host of different product combinations: you can have sativa THC, indica THC, as well as sativa CBD and indica CBD. The effects related to these terms are correctly attributed approximately 70 percent of the time, offering a good match for what people actually experience. But 30 percent of the time, individual differences yield a completely different effect. More recently, products are branded by their properties instead, like Energize or Relax.

Sativa products are generally stimulating, activating, and energizing. They are thought to deliver increased creativity, focus, and increased heart rate. For some people, that increase actually helps them calm down, just as Adderall can calm someone with ADHD. Yet for a great number of people, the activating effects of these cultivars can provoke anxiety. When I encourage people to approach cannabis with caution, the stimulating effect of sativa is at the top of the list of product categories that people should avoid. On the other hand, as people become familiar with the effects of THC, over time, the stimulating energy of sativa products can be uplifting and pleasant.

Indica products are much more complex. They are generally calming, quieting, sedating, relaxing. For many people, indica varieties help them go to sleep. For those who have restless leg syndrome or agitated thoughts, indica products generally quell those "activating" symptoms. It's not clear yet if so-called indica products actually have sedating properties, or if the hyper-focus that's created by the chemistry yields a muting of external/internal stimuli to create a relaxed atmosphere, just as the focused relaxation of meditation can bring.

Hybrid is the term used to describe plants that have qualities that seem to be between fully uplifting, activating effects and those that are more subduing. Hybrids are often formed by the joining, or hybridization, of multiple plants to cultivate desirable features of both into a new lineage of plant. Ironically, over the course of years of modern interbreeding of cannabis plants, it's now very rare to find so-called "purebred" products, and almost all products sold at dispensaries might be considered "hybrids" because in one way or another, most modern plants have borrowed horticultural advantages, and perhaps also sensation-producing qualities, from multiple cultivars.

The Most Common Dosing Mistakes

1. Taking too many edibles without waiting between them to see if there's going to be a delayed effect.
2. Not shopping at a place that's reputable: always look for a retailer's COA or buy from dispensaries whenever possible.
3. Giving up too soon. It's remarkably common for people to give up on cannabis therapies because of one bad experience. Trying new amounts, new products, different settings of consumption, or perhaps consuming with a supportive group of loved ones can make a world of difference in the effectiveness of cannabinoids.
4. Not ever taking a break. To avoid building a high tolerance, consider taking a cannabis break of one to two days, at least every two weeks. Daily use of cannabis can lead to increased dosage requirements, which is not harmful but can be costly. Changing the method of consumption, the type of products consumed, the dosage, and the frequency of products consumed can all help reduce developing tolerance.

5. Effective dosing of cannabis products is inextricable from the environment in which the cannabis is consumed. Coming at cannabis in the right frame of mind, and within supportive circumstances, can make or break the entire cannabis experience. While discovering your ideal situation, it also is critical to optimize your non-cannabis physiology, including sleep, hydration, exercise, and nutrition. You'll learn more about this concept, what I call *set and setting*, in the next chapter.

Finding Your Comfort Zone

Answer the following questions to help you start your product search:

1. *Have you enjoyed consuming cannabis products in the last few years?* If the answer is yes, you may be comfortable with a product that has a greater ratio of THC to CBD. If you've smoked cannabis in the past and you didn't enjoy it, try a CBD gummy or a candy or a tincture, or one with a lower ration of THC to CBD.

2. *Are euphoric effects attractive to you?* If the answer is yes, you will likely enjoy THC products or those with a greater ratio of THC to CBD.

3. *Would you like euphoria as an effect?* If the answer is yes, you will likely enjoy a pure THC choice.

4. *Would you like to avoid euphoria altogether?* If the answer is yes, you will likely enjoy CBD, CBG, or low-dose D8-THC choices.

5. *Would you like a shorter duration of action or a longer time course?* If shorter, you would benefit from inhaled options, carbonated drinks, topicals; if longer, you would like edibles.

6. *Would you prefer something calming/sedating/relaxing or something energizing and activating?* Indica options are supposed to be calming; sativa options are energizing and recommended unless you are inexperienced. Then I would propose hybrid options over sativa.

7. *Regarding edibles, are you looking for subtle effects or strong, impactful ones?* If subtle, start at lower doses, such as 2–3 mg. For a higher impact, and if

inexperienced, start with edibles closer to 5 mg, and if experienced, you may start higher.

8. *Are you typically sensitive to medicines or intoxicants (a little gets you a long way)?* You are very likely to experience the same hypersensitivity to cannabis. Start with the lowest dosages, and proceed patiently.

MEET DWAYNE

Dwayne is one of my favorite patients. He's a veteran who is struggling with PTSD. He experiences nightmares regularly and daily anxiety that has manifested as agoraphobia. Dwayne smoked marijuana in the past but hasn't touched it since he ended his military duty. He is frustrated with his inability to leave his home, and he contacted me after having a less than optimal experience with anti-anxiety medications.

I suggested that he start with low-dose, 2:1 CBD:THC gummies from a dispensary so that he could sleep better. I explained to him how to sign up at the dispensary, and that he may not feel anything for two or three days, but to keep at it: guided cannabis is a patient process.

Within a week Dwayne told me that he was already getting a better night's sleep. At the one-month checkup, we developed a new regimen to address both the nighttime and daytime issues. Although I typically don't recommend smoking cannabis, Dwayne's comfort and familiarity with it drove my initial approach to suggest that he could smoke cannabis during the daytime to quell his anxiety and use the gummies at night. I explained that, over time, I would strive to help Dwayne move away from smoking and toward safer, more efficient, and cost-effective alternatives.

When he reported back again three weeks later, Dwayne told me that his PTSD was remarkably better, not a nightly occurrence, but still there. During the day, his anxiety was no longer handicapping his activities. I assured Dwayne that he would be able to break from the grip of PTSD once and for all, and at that point, would no longer have to rely on cannabis to keep his anxiety in check.

Where to Shop

There is a gold standard of high-quality products for each point of purchase, and there are specific instances where I send my patients to each of these shopping options. For example, there's a cannabinoid called CBDA that I often recommend, yet it is only sold by a very limited number of manufacturers and can only be purchased from the online marketplace. In Massachusetts, where I live, medicinal products at the dispensary are less expensive than similar items found at the adult-use shops, and you can find more low-dose choices at dispensaries. However, that may not be the case where you live.

The State-Controlled Medical Dispensary

If you live in a state where you can purchase cannabis from a dispensary system, do so whenever possible, as it is always the safest option. Medical dispensaries carry pure, homogeneous, and reproducible products. They are mandated to provide exquisitely clean, nontoxic products, and products are tested rigorously.

Dispensaries are in the business of selling THC products, though some sell a premium CBD product that also contains 5 percent THC. Dispensaries can carry a wide variety of product types (edibles, oil, vape, flower, etc.), yet the actual number of products offered is typically much smaller than the totality of the online marketplace. However, if you find a product that you like at a medical dispensary, it's more likely that it will be in stock the next time you need it. What's more, you can often buy more of that product at a medical dispensary than you can buy from recreational outlets. The reason is that most states that have both medical dispensaries and adult-use shops are mandated to keep a certain portion of their sales for medical use: if they have a stockpile of products, they're required to offer those to medical patients first. Lastly, dispensaries can substantially discount medical cannabis because there is no tax on medicine, and states can heavily tax items that are "recreational." If privacy is a concern of yours, know that dispensaries follow HIPAA privacy protocols, which means that there are no records kept on purchases. The same is not true of the adult-use market, where they have the ability to track your purchasing habits along with your debit card information.

The rules for accessing dispensaries vary from state to state, yet for all states you will need a medical cannabis card from a doctor or other healthcare provider. Some states are more liberal with them than others. For example, some states limit the allowable diagnoses, while others give doctors freer rein. In some US states and a handful of other countries, medical dispensaries have pharmacists that can offer personalized advice. Pharmacists are rigorously trained healthcare specialists who understand the use, storage, and administration of medicine. They are experts at guiding patients on how to use medications and are well informed about potential adverse effects and concerning interactions.

The process of obtaining a medical card is similar in most regulated jurisdictions. Interested patients find a participating, preapproved medical provider either online, in participating medical facilities, or by word of mouth. Visits are conducted with varying degrees of traditional medical inquiry (forms, surveys) and medical interrogation, and occasionally supported by a formal data collection system. Most often, there is little to no emphasis on any objective laboratory testing, imaging, or a physical exam. If the medical provider believes the state's qualifying conditions have been met by the patient, and if there are no clear prohibitive factors, the patient will receive their medical card. Depending on the individual location and the certifying provider, this evaluation and approval process can cost anywhere from less than a hundred dollars up to several hundred.

Possessing a medical card opens a gateway to a whole world of products and opportunities that is closed to those without the license. Cannabis products sold in medical dispensaries are thoroughly lab tested and the potencies are guaranteed to be accurate. You won't have to worry about what you're using or if you can trust the quality. A medical card assures that you receive the best and finest quality every time. In several jurisdictions, there are also legal protections afforded to medical card holders. For instance, in several states, having a medical cannabis card provides strong support for someone fired on account of a positive cannabis test related to employment. A cannabis card is also necessary if you are looking for health insurance reimbursements or to make a workers' compensation claim.

CBD Stores

If you are looking for pure CBD products, these specialty shops are the way to go. They are physical stores that sell only CBD products—edibles, tinctures, creams, sucking candies in different concentrations—that are similar to what you can find online. You can also buy CBD products at gas stations, delis, mall carts, and in some states, at liquor stores. Besides CBD, these stores sometimes also sell products with CBN, Delta-8, and CBG. They may also carry products that combine CBD with melatonin (for better sleep), or terpenes sourced either from cannabis or other plants for scented products and added efficacy.

With so many products and so many places to shop, it can be difficult to determine the best place to purchase CBD products. As I've suggested before, check for an up-to-date COA. Most retailers who have a COA will prominently display it on the website and/or their products.

The Adult-Use (Recreational) Shop

The adult-use marketplace is typically geared toward products that are very high in THC or have only THC. Retail stores exist in states that have legalized adult-use or "recreational" cannabis. Regulations will vary from state to state. For example, in Massachusetts, the regulations are identical in medical dispensaries and adult-use stores, but that may not be the case where you live. Recreational retailers do not require a doctor's note, yet purchasers have to be over twenty-one years of age. Adult-use shops occasionally carry both CBD and THC products, including lower-dose THC options.

The Online Marketplace

The online marketplace for THC products is through state-sponsored dispensaries and can only be accessed with a medical card number. There is a plethora of CBD products online that come with lab testing COAs, including Delta-8-THC (which is made from CBD). All CBD products are completely accessible.

What's Next

In the next chapter, you will discover how to use the information you've learned so far to create your own cannabis products, both edibles and topicals. If you can't find the exact product you're looking for, you do have the ability to create exactly what you want from the best available ingredients.

CHAPTER 4

Do-It-Yourself Products, Edibles, and Topicals

The future of the cannabis commercial ecosystem will contain a rainbow of selection. The industry is maturing cautiously, and at a piecemeal pace. One day, you will be able to pick and choose between products that provide exactly the effects you want, including specific botanicals, flavonoids, and terpenes. As of this writing, those nuances that may provide real relief are often absent, leaving consumers with the shallow decision of the presence or absence of euphoric effects.

The following instructions provide ways for you to hack the products that are available at dispensaries and online to meet your specific needs for edibles, topicals, and more.

First, to Decarboxylate Your Cannabis . . . or Not

Decarboxylating, or "decarbing," occurs when the dehydrated cannabis flower you buy at dispensaries is heated just enough to transform its nascent compounds into active forms. For instance, heated THC is intensely euphoric, while in the preheated state, the innate plant isn't. Until recently, many believed that because decarboxylated forms of THC are more euphoric, its preheated form was inactive. This has been disproven, and not only are the pre-decarboxylated forms active in the body, but in some cases, these so-called "acid forms" may have their own advantages over heated forms. Consuming unheated cannabis (mixing the raw plant form into smoothies, for example) has been studied for treatments including inflammation and nausea. Heating partially, at lower temperatures through decarbing, can give you the advantages of both forms.

The most common way to decarb cannabis is to first choose a flower product that features a variety of colors, visible crystals, and hairs. Break the flower into small pieces, placing it on a sheet pan and baking it in an oven at 220 degrees for twenty-five minutes. It is also recommended to drop the temperature lower, and bake a little bit longer, to preserve more terpenes (some of them evaporate at higher temperatures), which in turn will give you a broader variety of medicinally active compounds. Once you have decarbed the cannabis, you are ready to use it to make an edible, following the recipes in this chapter.

While ingesting cannabis is discrete, the preparations aren't as much. Decarbing will create a strong aroma of cannabis in your kitchen. For those who are concerned about the aroma, there are products that neutralize the odors from decarboxylation, as well as from carrying or consuming cannabis.

Upgrading Cannabis Flower

An easier way to hack cannabis plants to produce the desired effect you may be looking for is to combine them with products that have known characteristics. For instance, using a sealable plastic storage container, put cannabis flower inside, along with a few drops of a desired terpene or flavonoid. Seal the bag and let it sit overnight until the cannabis absorbs some of the additive's medicinal properties.

Terpenes are often sold as essential oils in various formulations, densities, and degrees of good manufacturing: look for ones that are safe to consume. Please note the safety and appropriate-use documentation for any/all products purchased from a terpene manufacturer prior to consuming, as many terpenes are sold at very high concentrations, and they can be toxic if not properly diluted.

Understanding Boiling Points

You can tap into a wide variety of medicinal qualities held within the cannabis plant by accessing the exact cannabinoids, terpenes, and flavonoids that you require. Right now, the commercial ecosystem cannot effectively extract all of these compounds efficiently or affordably. Instead of waiting for industry to catch up with your needs, you can extract these same compounds at home by boiling cannabis flower at specific temperatures and then vaporizing the medicine of your choice.

Different components of cannabis have different boiling point temperatures (see chart on the following page). Many vaporizers sold today can target specific temperatures. By adjusting the temperature of your vaporizer, you can control which compounds (cannabinoids, terpenoids, and flavonoids) rise into the air (typically up into a mouthpiece or an inflatable bag to capture the gas), so you can select the medicinal qualities you need. Then, you can experiment with dosage and frequency of the newly vaporized product in exactly the same way you would experiment with any other cannabis product.

Prior to heating the plant to the temperature that will aerosolize your desired compound, consider heating to a slightly lower temperature for a few seconds, without inhaling, before moving up. This way, the molecules that vaporize at lower temperatures can be exhausted first, and the result after raising the heat slightly will be a higher density of those desirable components that had not yet boiled off at lower temperatures. For example, my patient Eric, who suffers from migraines, sets his vaporizer at specific degrees using the same cannabis flower product and gets dramatically different outcomes. First, he heats his flower to 250° Fahrenheit, so that the acids on the raw flower, and CO_2, are being gassed off.

On the weekends, he heats cannabis flower to 250° and then to 315°, at which point he will be inhaling more Delta-9-THC than was available to him from his initial purchase. This compound helps him control his migraines while providing an increased opportunity for sleep. It also comes with a more euphoric effect that doesn't compromise his job. Each time Eric vaporizes, he is not extracting the full contents of the cannabinoids, so the 315° boiling point product can last two or three sessions. However, with each subsequent session, the result tastes more like burnt popcorn. This is why it is best to dial into the lowest boiling points for your needs first and raise the temperature as needed. Then, after three sessions, he can use the remaining cannabis for making THC edibles that still contain potent compounds.

If he didn't need all three sessions over the weekend, the leftover flower in the vaporizer from his weekend use now already has more CBD than the raw flower he originally purchased. If he then sets the vaporizer to 338°, he will be able to extract more CBD (which boils between 320–356° Fahrenheit), which allows him to medicate during the workday and feel more lucid.

BOILING POINT TEMPERATURE	CANNABINOID	REPORTED USE
126° F	Cannabigerol—CBG	Non-euphoric: antibacterial, antidepressant, antifungal, anti-inflammatory, antimicrobial, anti-neoplastic (tumors), bone stimulant, bowel relaxant, mood stabilizer. Provides relief for skin irritation (eczema, psoriasis, acne), anxiety, glaucoma, insomnia, pain, gastrointestinal diseases.
220° F (Range: 140°–257° F)	Tetrahydrocannabinolic Acid—THCA	Euphoric: anti-inflammatory, appetite stimulant, anti-neoplastic, bowel relaxant, neurostimulant, anti-convulsant. Provides relief for asthma, cough, glaucoma, insomnia, nausea, pain, muscle spasm, seizure, swelling, multiple sclerosis, diabetes, IBS, Crohn's disease. Higher doses associated with hunger, paranoia, elevated pulse rate, immune modulation, sedation.

BOILING POINT TEMPERATURE	CANNABINOID	REPORTED USE
248° F	Cannabidiolic Acid—CBDA	Euphoric: anti-inflammatory, appetite stimulant, anti-neoplastic, bowel relaxant, neurostimulant, anti-convulsant. Provides relief for asthma, cough, glaucoma, insomnia, nausea, pain, muscle spasm, seizure, swelling, multiple sclerosis, diabetes, IBS, Crohn's disease. Higher doses associated with hunger, paranoia, elevated pulse rate, immune modulation, sedation.
.248° F	Cannabichromenic Acid—CBCA	Euphoric: anti-inflammatory, appetite stimulant, anti-neoplastic, bowel relaxant, neurostimulant, anti-convulsant. Provides relief for asthma, cough, glaucoma, insomnia, nausea, pain, muscle spasm, seizure, swelling, multiple sclerosis, diabetes, IBS, Crohn's disease. Higher doses associated with hunger, paranoia, elevated pulse rate, immune modulation, sedation.

BOILING POINT TEMPERATURE	CANNABINOID	REPORTED USE
315° F	Tetrahydrocannabinol—Delta-9-THC	Euphoric: anti-inflammatory, appetite stimulant, anti-neoplastic, bowel relaxant, neurostimulant, anti-convulsant. Provides relief for asthma, cough, glaucoma, insomnia, nausea, pain, muscle spasm, seizure, swelling, multiple sclerosis, diabetes, IBS, Crohn's disease. Higher doses associated with hunger, paranoia, elevated pulse rate, immune modulation, sedation.
338° F (Range: 320°–356° F)	Cannabidiol—CBD	Non-euphoric: antidepressant, anti-inflammatory, antioxidant, anti-neoplastic. Provides relief for anxiety (strong), arthritis, elevated heart rate, insomnia, muscle spasm, nausea, pain, seizure. Supports lipid, blood-sugar level stabilization, immune modulation, neuroprotection.
349° F (Range: 347°–352° F)	Delta 8-Tetrahydro-cannabinol—D8-THC	Mildly euphoric: antidepressant, antioxidant, anti-neoplastic, appetite stimulant, neuroprotective, neurostimulant, reduces toxins. Provides relief for anxiety, nausea, pain, glaucoma, insomnia.

BOILING POINT TEMPERATURE	CANNABINOID	REPORTED USE
365° F	Cannabinol—CBN	Mildly euphoric: antibacterial, anti-inflammatory, appetite stimulant, neuroprotective. Provides relief for ALS symptoms, asthma, nausea, pain, seizures; sedative, skin soothing (eczema, psoriasis, acne), IBS, hypertension.
385° F	Cannabielsoin—CBE	Mildly euphoric: antidepressant, mood stabilizer, anti-tumor. Provides relief for anxiety, pain; with linalool or limonene: sedative, potentiates immunity.
428° F	Tetrahydrocannabi-varin—THCV	Mildly euphoric: antibacterial, appetite suppressant, increases metabolism, increases short-term memory, improves speech impairment, neuroprotective, anti-convulsant. Provides relief for nausea, pain, seizures, acne, Parkinson's disease.
428° F	Cannabichromene—CBC	Non-euphoric: antioxidant, anti-neoplastic. Provides relief for pain and swelling.

Make Your Own Tinctures

It's easy to make tinctures at home. Once it is made, you can use a serial dilutions technique whereby you cut a concentrated solution in half repeatedly until you get to a dose that is too weak to be useful. Then, backtrack to the previous level of dilution: this will be your ideal dosage.

Alcohol-Based Tinctures

You will need:

+ ⅛ oz. raw flower-form cannabis
+ 10 oz. Everclear or other ultra-high-proof alcohol (the higher the proof, the better)

Instructions:

1. Preheat the oven to 240° F.
2. Spread ground cannabis on a baking sheet. Decarboxylate the cannabis in the oven for twenty-five to thirty minutes.
3. Remove from the oven. Pour the contents into a glass jar with a tight-fitting lid.
4. Pour the alcohol into the jar until it covers the cannabis. Cover the jar tightly and shake it until the contents are well mixed. Store the jar in a warm, dark place overnight (or longer).
5. After twenty-four hours, strain the mixture through a cheesecloth into a measuring cup. Store your tincture in medicine bottles with a dropper for easiest use.
6. Consider sending your tincture to a laboratory to determine the specific concentrations of active ingredients. They will send you a report so that you can have insight into the chemical makeup of your tincture.

Infusions or Oil-Based Tinctures

An oil-based tincture is properly referred to as an *infusion*.

To make one at home you will need:

+ ¼ oz. raw flower-form cannabis
+ 8 oz. grapeseed oil (or other purified oil of your choosing)

Instructions:

1. Preheat the oven to 240° F.

2. Spread ground cannabis on a baking sheet. Decarboxylate the cannabis in the oven for twenty-five to thirty minutes.

3. Remove from the oven, and divide the cannabis evenly into two jars with tight-fitting lids. Divide the oil into each jar and seal tightly.

4. Place the jars into a slow cooker and cover with boiling water so that the jars are fully submerged. Set the slow cooker to "warm" and let cook for four hours. Using oven mitts or kitchen tongs, pull the jars out once an hour and give them a good shake. After four hours, remove the jars and let them cool.

5. Line a large funnel with four layers of cheesecloth and place it over a measuring cup. Pour the liquid through the cheesecloth. Then, transfer the oil into smaller tincture bottles. Let the contents fully cool before use. If the oil-based or alcohol-based tinctures taste unpleasant, try freezing them before consuming or adding your favorite flavors such as cinnamon, mint, citrus, or lavender (all of which happen to be terpenes also produced in cannabis). Holding your nose to block airflow can also help mask unpleasant tastes.

Use Water-Soluble Tinctures for Edibles

Alcohol-based tinctures will easily mix with water and other liquids, while oil-based tinctures won't, and will therefore limit your ability to consume the full dose. However, oil-based tinctures can be made water-soluble at home. These tinctures are available in the marketplace, but they can be difficult to find. Simply blend the existing infusion vigorously with an emulsifier, such as gum arabic or Acacia senegal. Emulsifying the cannabis-based oil with gum arabic makes it easy to incorporate the product into any water-based cocktail recipe. Emulsifying your tincture with gum arabic and adding a non-cannabis liquid will slightly dilute the known dose of the cannabis oil, introducing some uncertainty about its strength, but also increasing the opportunity to mix desirable flavors and potentially more appealing foods or drinks.

Make Your Own Edibles

The base of edibles is generally a fat, such as butter, oil, or mayonnaise, that has been infused with a cannabis product. You can use an existing distillate, tincture, or other forms of cannabis concentrates in the kitchen to incorporate cannabinoids into the culinary experience. Kief, wax, shatter, budder, RSO, and other forms of sticky concentrate all offer unique attributes that may be appealing for cooking. Some are comprised of more inert waxy components, while others have been formed to shed their neutral waxes in favor of their medicinally active inner components. Oil-based cannabis products like tinctures and distillates are great for baking and cooking because they can be used as the fat or oil required in recipes. There are also concentrate drops that have already been emulsified that you can squeeze into your favorite beverage.

Cooking with cannabis is an easy way for you to incorporate your treatment into your diet. Depending on the method and process of their manufacture, some concentrate products are mild in flavor, while some can be very strong and pungent. You can also purchase a tincture that features a terpene such as limonene, which will smell and taste citrusy, and enhance the taste of an edible, like a citrus-flavored dressing.

Some dispensaries sell grapeseed or other cooking oils that are already infused with cannabis. You can also add cannabis to recipes by creating your own cannabis-based oil, mayonnaise, or butter. This can be done adding a known concentration of cannabis product to an existing dietary fat, and this requires careful experimentation and accurate recordkeeping to achieve consistent dosages and reproducible effects. For instance, you can make several formulations of a cannabis oil or mayonnaise at the same time using different amounts of concentrate, increasing the dosage until you hit on the desired effect. The goal is to create a consistent, reproducible product that meets your unique needs, so you know you will be taking the same dose every time. To test, make a single serving and be sure to eat or drink the entire portion.

To make cannabis butter, add concentrate or decarbed cannabis into melted butter at a 1:1 ratio in a saucepan over medium heat. Add an equal amount of water to butter. Make sure that you are constantly stirring, creating as homogeneous a mixture as possible. If a product lacks uniformity, you will be creating wildly different doses, and it would be impossible to reproduce desirable effects.

Then, strain through a cheesecloth into a short jar with a lid. Refrigerate until the liquid becomes a solid butter. Remove any excess water. After you infuse butter with cannabis, you can spread it directly on toast or use it to make baked goods. For instance, if your favorite brownie recipe calls for ½ cup of butter, you can fully replace that component with ½ cup of cannabis-infused butter, or partially replace some of the ½ cup, depending on how strong you need the end product to be. You can also add a few drops of concentrated oil to the ½ cup of regular butter, which will provide some cannabis but lower the dose even further.

Make Your Own Cannabis Pills, Capsules, and Tablets

Pills, capsules, and tablets can be easily made at home with known doses of raw cannabis products, such as concentrates, distillates, and tinctures. Dividing known portions of these concentrated ingredients into small products provides a simple, discrete method of consumption. Empty capsules can be purchased from online retailers, and they can even accommodate dietary sensitivities, including vegetarian, vegan, gluten-free, and gelatin-free varieties.

Make Your Own Topicals

Lotions, salves, lubricants, and balms are commonly referred to as *topicals*. These are cannabis-infused products that are applied to the skin and offer localized pain relief. Euphoric results are rarely associated with topicals because the THC (and other cannabinoids) do not penetrate into the bloodstream in sufficient amounts to bring on strong downstream effects. However, topicals can be surprisingly effective and fast-acting locally, as they quickly and easily cross the skin membranes and have powerful effects on local tissues, including skin, muscle, blood vessels, and nerves.

Unfortunately, the bulk of the topicals sold in today's markets do not contain as much cannabis as they should, regardless of whether it is CBD- or

THC-dominant. And dispensaries carry a small fraction of all the potential therapeutic products they could. If you can't find the topical you are searching for, you can purchase any of three categories of products at dispensaries—flower, tincture, or concentrate—and make individualized cannabis topicals at home, using existing products that you can buy in a regular drugstore to serve as the base.

Basically, all lotions are a mixture of water and oil in varying ratios. You can choose your base product by your needs or personal preferences. I have found success with every thickness, from creamy balms all the way to the thinnest lotions. A petroleum jelly product, like Vaseline, is 100 percent oil, which means that it is 100 percent occlusive. Using it as a base for a cannabis balm applied to the skin would help avoid evaporation of the topical, and further assist with effective penetration into the skin and deeper tissues. On the other end of the spectrum, there are lotions that are mostly water, which would be good for tissues that are sensitive to oily textures, including areas around the eyes, within the nose, at some joints, and in/around genitalia or anal tissues. You can use pure coconut oil as a base for topicals, like lubricants, and even for applying cannabinoids to the scalp (for moisturization or for its anti-inflammatory action).

The process to create cannabinoid topicals is simple and takes less than an hour to complete.

Basic Lotion Recipe

1. In a glass jar, mix 3–4 grams of cannabis concentrate (shatter is preferable to wax, which is preferable to kief) or a highly concentrated tincture or oil with ½ to ¾ cup of any body lotion. Seal the jar tightly, and place it inside a saucepan full of boiling water. Let the jar heat up for about forty minutes, ensuring that the saucepan has a steady supply of boiling water to avoid drying out.
2. Remove the jar from the boiling water, and with kitchen gloves on, shake the jar vigorously for several minutes.
3. Let the evenly distributed mixture re-congeal in a refrigerator before using.

Make Your Own Balm

If you want to make a thicker balm directly from flower, you will need the following ingredients:

+ ¼ oz. ground cannabis in its raw-flower form
+ 1½ cups coconut oil
+ ⅓ cup beeswax

Instructions:

1. Preheat the oven to 240° F.
2. Spread dried, ground cannabis on a baking sheet. Decarboxylate the cannabis in the oven for twenty-five to thirty minutes.
3. Meanwhile, place the coconut oil in a saucepan or double boiler over low heat and stir continuously until it melts.
4. Remove the cannabis from the oven and mix it into the coconut oil. Over low heat, continue to stir the mixture for twenty to twenty-five minutes.
5. Remove from heat and pour the mixture through a cheesecloth into a clean jar.
6. Place the beeswax into a second jar and heat it in a double boiler until it is melted. When it is melted, transfer it to the container of infused coconut oil. Mix thoroughly and allow the product to cool completely before using it.

Make Your Own Personal Lubricant

For men, cannabis-infused lubricants increase blood flow to the penis and heighten sensations. For women, they cause more intense orgasms and full-body sexual experiences, while offering an antidote to vaginal dryness and soothing other forms of vaginal discomfort. The following recipe uses a coconut oil base, which yields a thick and long-lasting lubricant, but it's not compatible with latex condoms.

To make the lubricant, follow the tincture recipe on page 90, substituting 8 oz. coconut oil. Or, if you are starting with concentrate, add 4–6 grams of concentrate to 8 oz. of coconut oil.

What's Next

In the next chapter, you will learn how different products interact with your body, which will depend not only on how you are feeling but the "set-and-setting" differences that impact you. Both our internal health and mindset, as well as our external setting, can impact our experience of cannabis. Taking the same product during occasions when you're experiencing different moods may produce completely different experiences. Similarly, cannabis consumed in a physically comfortable setting will likely create a very different experience than cannabis consumed in awkward or perilous circumstances. Exploring a handful of different types of products, and using them across a variety of different moods and conditions, may help you see how different circumstances may be a better match for some products over others. What's more, your body will react differently to different types of products; not all cannabis feels or acts the same, and in some cases, the differences are profound!

CHAPTER 5

Starting Your Guided Cannabis Journey

Here is a subset of people who have initial success with cannabis, only to later feel like they hit a wall in their recovery. More often than not, I believe the reason they are not fully satisfied is that they neglected to put the rest of their wellness house in order: if you expect lasting results, you can't fix one domain of health and not address the others. A less than optimal environment, which includes the way you live your life as well as the quality of your surroundings, can strongly impact your experience with cannabis. Understanding your internal and external environments, or what I call your "set and setting," is just as important as choosing between THC or CBD products.

Optimize Your Environment

The medical community has known for some time that optimizing one's environment improved health outcomes, yet we didn't know exactly why this idea was true. It's now believed that there are two important theories at play, and the endocannabinoid system is integral in both. The first is the theory of epigenetics, which posits that your genetic code is not strictly your destiny. Even if you come from a long line of people with certain health conditions like heart disease, obesity, and diabetes, the way you live your life now can influence whether the genes that predispose you to those diseases are turned on or off. Maintaining a healthy diet, exercising regularly, and reducing stress have long been thought of ways to modulate epigenetic expression. Cannabis can play an important role in optimizing each of these environmental factors.

Secondly, the biochemical roots of feelings like contentment and satisfaction are influenced by the endocannabinoid system, and cannabis, as well as environmental factors like exercise, eating healthfully, and lowering stress, are all ways to bolster the system's activity. If you can maintain an attitude of satisfaction and joy, you will naturally create a fusion of medicine and experience that is more harmonious, and thus, more effective.

In this chapter, I'll review the different facets of a typical environment, so that you can pay careful attention and amplify lifestyle choices that will positively affect your health. If you do so before you address specific health complaints, you'll find that cannabis actually works better. For instance, a hangover is very likely to occur if you are consuming cannabis while not adequately hydrated; it can be avoided if you are already in the habit of drinking plenty of water each day. Similarly, you may experience different effects from cannabis when it is consumed with specific foods, and the healthier your diet is, the better results you'll see.

Upgrade Food and Nutrition

In the same way that we are just beginning to understand how the endocannabinoid system works, the overall role that the digestive system plays in total body health is not yet completely understood. Whereas once it was believed that the gastrointestinal system existed merely to absorb nutrients and fluids, we now understand the realities of a true mind-gut connection, as well as the importance of the gut microbiome in terms of enhancing the body's immune and metabolic ecosystems. There is a growing recognition in the scientific community that the foods we eat play an essential role in our health and happiness, and that macronutrients, vitamins, and minerals are part of a unique communication system that can augment cannabinoids and terpenoid molecules.

The easiest diet to follow is the one that features the foods you love without feeling deprived, which is why I don't recommend a diet that is high in one macronutrient—whether proteins, carbs, or fats—over another. In general, a balanced diet is best. Choose minimally processed foods that look like their original source: a variety of fresh and colorful fruits and vegetables, lean meats, poultry, fish and seafood, healthy fats and oils rich in polyunsaturated and monounsaturated fatty acids, with a selection of complex carbohydrates. Limit foods and drinks that are high in added sugars (including soft drinks and alcoholic beverages), saturated fat, and table salt.[1] Most of us can meet our vitamin and mineral requirements through good food, though some may need to enhance their diet with nutritional supplements. For example, if you have restless leg syndrome, you may have been told that you have a deficiency in iron, vitamin D, or magnesium. If your vitamin B or C is inadequate, you can have serious physical and mental health consequences. What's more, without the proper levels of basic vitamins and minerals, cannabis therapies can have unpredictable effects. Your healthcare provider can perform a nutritional analysis and tailor supplement suggestions to your specific needs.

It is good to please one's taste buds; it is better to please your other organs, too. Following these guidelines can reduce your risk of chronic diseases, including cardiovascular disease, type 2 diabetes, certain cancers (breast, colon, and rectum), and osteoporosis. And simply cleaning up your diet can help you lose weight; if you are looking for significant weight loss, consider reducing portion sizes. Interestingly, the clinical data following people who consume cannabis regularly shows that they have better weight control than people who don't consume cannabis.[2]

Cannabis will operate most efficiently when your digestive system is steady and satisfied. Satisfaction is undeniably an individual experience and a unique judgment. For some, nutritious food choices make for a meal to be satisfying. For others, a particularly pleasing taste brings exhilaration and a sense of being content. Beyond personal preferences, however, there are some features of the interaction between food and cannabis that apply across individual differences.

First, you don't want to be hungry before beginning a cannabis experience. Placing your attention on hunger creates thought patterns that can easily derail an otherwise pleasant cannabis experience, because it is distracting. Yet taking cannabis on a completely full stomach will delay the body's interaction with edibles and tinctures by as much as three hours, depending on the amount and types of foods blocking the way forward. My advice: go for the Goldilocks approach—not too hungry that you are annoyed, but not too full that you feel bloated or uncomfortable.

Certain types of foods will also influence the effects of the cannabis. Foods that alter the body's metabolism of energy (sugars vs. oils/fats vs. proteins) or inhibit or amplify other biological pathways (inflammation vs. hormonal vs. circadian biochemistry) also reshape the way cannabis is absorbed and functions within the biological ecosystem. For instance, our body has a unique system to absorb nutrient-dense foods, like dietary fats and oils; the body creates a *chylomicron*, a particle that transports fat with priority through the digestive tract. Foods that are rich in oils, then, absorb cannabinoids and are effective tools that can be used to speed absorption and/or lengthen the duration of action. This is why I often recommend chocolate cannabis edibles made from butter or oil over sugar gummies, because the effects tend to last longer, with less dramatic energetic highs and lows. Another easy way to increase healthy fats and oils is simply switching your salad dressing to one that is oil-based before or after dosing. You can also make your own cannabis butter to use in baking recipes (see chapter four).

Maintain Adequate Hydration

Suboptimal hydration is one of the most common sources of discomfort associated with cannabis. One of the most prominent side effects of cannabis is that it dries out tissues throughout the body, causing dry mouth, dry eyes, drier stool, and so on. These annoyances can be remedied by drinking more water, or increasing your intake of fruits and vegetables, which are naturally hydrating. Regardless of cannabis usage, I typically recommend that adults drink to optimal hydration, at least 2 liters of water every day. You can tell if you are adequately hydrated if your urine is clear rather than darker yellow (although the first urination of the day doesn't count: when you wake up in the morning, your first urine can be yellowish).

Cannabis should move fluidly through your body via the bloodstream in an even dosage, as opposed to a compressed or high-octane dosage. Without proper hydration, you will have a higher concentration of cannabis in your blood vessels, and you will feel its effects more strongly and more rapidly. Other side effects of inadequate hydration and cannabis include dizziness, light-headedness, a hangover, experiences of extremely intense euphoria, heart palpitations, stomach upsets, and excessive anxiety or appetite stimulation.

When you are dosing cannabis, make sure to drink water before, during, and after; especially after. Any natural source of hydration is good, the only caveat being fruit juices high in vitamin C—like orange juice or grapefruit juice—which seem to act as competitors in the endocannabinoid system, and may also more quickly clear cannabinoids. If you are drinking citrus juice on some days and not others, you're likely to have an inconsistent experience with the effects of cannabis: best to choose a different juice or flavored water. There are cannabis beverages, or you can put cannabis concentrate into a water-soluble drink. However, it's not known if these beverages count toward your hydration total. If they are made with sugars and other concentrated additives, they may have a dehydrating effect.

Adopt an Exercise Program

Exercise is an important component of wellness, especially when you are using cannabis as medicine. Having a healthy exercise routine not only strengthens muscles that process cannabinoids and other nutrition, but it also helps stimulate the release of cannabinoids that are stored in fat cells throughout the body— exercise squeezes fat cells, and the cannabis that is stored inside gets expunged. At the same time, exercise also fosters the release of other neurotransmitters (norepinephrine, dopamine, serotonin) into the bloodstream that are thought to reinforce feelings of well-being and peak performance, such as a runner's high. Therefore, when people are exercising, they can create a naturally higher endocannabinoid state.

Whether it's enhanced attention or just the right dose of relaxing chemistry, athletes as well as casual fitness fans seem to benefit from cannabis as part of the routine. I've found that my patients who use cannabis while exercising feel like they can push through their normal limits and get more out of their workout. For some, this seems to be a matter of enhanced focus. It's common for my patients to describe feeling less distracted, more curious, and more motivated by body sensations rather than discouraged by them. In the case of exercise that may be physically challenging or uncomfortable, the pleasant chemistry of cannabis can easily and quickly counterbalance the temporary strain.

There are no limits to what is considered to be the right amount of healthy exercise, and most adults need at least 150 minutes of exercise per week. No matter what your age, the best exercise programs include both aerobic exercise that gets your heart pumping and body sweating, and strength training to support muscle and bone health. You don't have to pump iron at the gym or buy into the latest fads for stationary bikes. A solid exercise program can be as simple as walking briskly enough so that you are unable to carry a conversation. Talk to your healthcare provider before you start any exercise program, and let them know you are following a cannabis therapy protocol. A knowledgeable cannabis physician can point you toward the specific products that will help you with exercise, which will be covered in chapter eleven.

Identify Stressors and Your Go-To Response to Them

Many of my patients do not fully understand what is causing their physical and emotional discomfort. Taking a clear look at what stressors you may be dealing with, and how they are affecting your quality of life, is an activity worth pursuing. The way you feel about your job, your home life, and yourself will each have a meaningful impact on your general well-being. Then, think about the ways you're already responding to these stressors. If you're drinking a lot of alcohol, getting poor sleep, or eating junky foods, it's not just the stress that is having an impact on your health. By identifying your current coping mechanisms, and swapping them out for healthier ones, you may be better able to handle your stress and improve your overall health. The activities that go well with cannabis—including meditation, listening to music, exercising, sleeping, laughing, and playing—are all practices that support, if not outright define, a healthy lifestyle. Engaging in any of these activities can be an antidote to daily stressors and offer new opportunities for decompression.

For instance, a meditation or mindfulness practice helps you to become centered, present, and focused. It can help alleviate the burden of rumination and allow you to see the joy and beauty in the moment. Cannabis, which inherently presents the brain with opportunities to discover novelty, for creating new connections, and strengthening old connections that have been lost, can be a very effective tool during meditation. Its ability to aid in forgetfulness can synergistically amplify the therapeutic benefits of meditation, leading to greater empathy, sympathy, and compassion for yourself and others, and above all, offer a powerful magnetism to the ever-fleeting present moment.

Cannabis Isn't a Coping Mechanism

Some people use cannabis as a crutch to help them avoid the difficulties of life, because it offers such an effective way to relax. So it would be no surprise that, beyond your specific medical needs, you may find that cannabis becomes part of your process for relaxing. While I'm certainly not opposed to this, be aware that cannabis can improve your stress levels, but only for a short period of time. While you may find an otherwise elusive sense of calmness when consuming cannabis, if you have consistent, even chronic stressors, no amount of cannabis product alone can overcome them.

Cannabis use is not a free pass for avoiding your issues. If you forget to practice the often-difficult skills of engaging in life, you're going to suffer even more. That's why I recommend that you practice living with stressors without cannabis—to see how you can alleviate those difficulties on your own. All of us need to develop effective coping skills to help us manage the ups and downs of life. Asking a friend for help, taking time off, exercise, meditation, getting better sleep, and upgrading your diet—all of the ways we discussed improving your environment in this chapter—are proven strategies that will work now and over time. Cannabis won't have the long-term benefits that these factors, as well as improving your interpersonal skills, will provide.

If you are faced with a life that seems too complicated, or too burdensome to navigate alone, ask for help. Think about it: If you're open to taking this first leap into a cutting-edge opportunity in medicine, isn't it also time that you ask for the help you need from others?

MEET JIMMY

Jimmy came to see me when he was sixty years old and 110 pounds over-weight. He was completely stressed out: he had left his job in the restaurant industry because of the pandemic and was still searching for a new career. He was already taking a boatload of medicines because his doctor told him that otherwise he would have a heart attack; he had a strong family history of heart disease. He was also taking medicine to treat his diabetes, and his doctor recently had added on insulin. This last prescription was the final straw. Jimmy told me that he doesn't like taking so many medicines because he doesn't want to be "like his parents," who took a lot of medicines. At this point he was desperate to try something new.

Jimmy wanted to talk to me about cannabis therapies that could poten-tially help him lose weight in the hopes that he could get his health back on track. He knew he didn't want to smoke cannabis because he had kids at home. He wanted to know if there were other options available to him. I explained that Jimmy's regimen would be under his full control. We reviewed the basics of the formulations and the products he could choose from to find something that would appeal to him. We picked a CBD-dominant tincture for the days that he needs to be more motivated to exercise, and a dispensary flower rich in THCV (known to suppress appetite and improve insulin pro-duction) for relaxation following high-stress days, or for when he was feeling overwhelmed or needed to sleep better. He could also take them together to help him improve his anxiety and his exercise tolerance.

Three months later we had a telehealth appointment, and I could tell that Jimmy was noticeably well rested. He was excited to let me know that he was starting to lose weight for the first time in years. He was able to exercise more frequently each week, and was in a lot less pain.

A year after he started his guided cannabis therapy, Jimmy had lost a total of forty pounds and was sleeping well consistently. Better still, his blood glucose levels were getting better every month. He had already adjusted his insulin routine twice because he required less medicine.

Adapting Your Physical Space

Having appropriate ambient sensory input is critical to a successful experience with cannabis for the same reasons as eating the right amount of food: you don't want to be bothered by negative distractions. Cannabis amplifies the intensity of our brain circuitry and allows us to extend its boundaries. When you're thinking happy thoughts, when you're feeling comfortable, cannabis will amplify that experience. When your circuits of discomfort are activated, the very same types of cannabis that energize happiness will be equally effective amplifying negative emotions.

Pay attention to what your room looks like, what your environment looks like, because the more comfortable you are in your space, the better you will feel. Do you have a favorite chair or comfortable spot in your home? Are you cozy in your bed, or is that just the place to conk out? Are you overstimulated with bright lights or loud noises? Are you unnecessarily chilly or warm? All of these states can set off neural circuits of discomfort that influence cannabis effectiveness. It's like the difference between staying in a hospital room surrounded by sterile, uninviting materials and being in a room with a homemade quilt, photos of your loved ones around, and a comfortable pillow. It's a totally different experience, and comfort begets more comfort, which in turn begets improved health.

Being around people with whom you're comfortable is also important. Conversations that are reciprocal and agreeable will enhance your cannabis experience, compared to discussions with disagreements or controversy. My clinical data following more than 16,000 CED Clinic patients found that when compared with patients who kept their cannabis consumption to themselves, those who were open about their cannabis consumption were significantly more likely to achieve success.

Talk to Your Healthcare Provider About Medical Cannabis

Bringing up the topic of medical cannabis with your healthcare provider can feel intimidating and anxiety-provoking. Many people fear being judged or worry that they'll face consequences for admitting they have used cannabis in the past or want to use it in the future. Let's lay that worry to rest: just like all medical information, your cannabis use remains part of the private conversation between you and your healthcare provider. National privacy laws, such as HIPAA, equally apply for medical cannabis healthcare providers as they do for all other types of healthcare providers.

Feeling comfortable speaking to your healthcare provider about medical cannabis can be daunting, but it shouldn't dissuade you from seeking help. If you are nervous about approaching your provider about your plans, here are some tips on how to initiate the conversation:

+ Think about your real goals. Write down reasons why you feel medical cannabis may be right for you.
+ Bring your notes to your next appointment, and try something like, "I want to learn more about medical cannabis," or "I believe medical cannabis may be a good treatment option for me—do you agree?"
+ Bring a family member or friend who has experience with medical cannabis to your appointment. This may help you feel more comfortable speaking with your healthcare provider.
+ Ask your primary care provider if they are comfortable with and knowledgeable about cannabis.

Evaluate Your Existing Medications

Before starting any new medical protocol, it's a good idea to evaluate your existing medications to see whether they're actually necessary, and whether they're contributing to a positive quality of life. Many people take multiple medications prescribed by different healthcare providers, who each may not know what other prescribers have recommended. Clinicians often assume that medications don't meaningfully interact with food or other medications or supplements, and it can be alarmingly common for clinicians to tack on additional medications to a regimen without considering what the patient may already be taking. The result is that many people take medications that they do not need, and they experience effects and interactions that elude their prescribing physicians. Prescription medications, over-the-counter therapies, as well as supplements and nutraceuticals, can affect each other, and patients often suffer the consequences.

Cannabis, like its fruit and vegetable relatives, is compatible with most medicines, because it interacts with the same systems and pathways in the body that traditional medicines do. However, freely flowing cannabis will act on whatever tissues it interacts with, and any medications that affect the brain's chemistry will be affected by cannabis. For instance, antidepressant medications typically exert their effects at the serotonin-signaling neuron junctions in the brain. Cannabis activates these same junctions, albeit in a slightly different manner, and the result of the combination of antidepressant and cannabis medication is typically a synergistic boosting of the effects of both medications. This means that while you are taking antidepressants, you may find that you need a smaller cannabis dosage to achieve the effect you are looking for. And the presence of cannabis means that you may also be able to use less medication to achieve the same pharmaceutical goals.

The part of the body that processes medicines, namely the liver, also breaks down cannabis. When liver enzymes are preparing one medicine, they are not available to degrade cannabis. The result is that the cannabis you consumed may take another turn through the system circulation, and the effect tends to be more potent. Conversely, when the liver's acting on cannabis, other medicines that are typically degraded also tend to be more potent. Some medications, like blood thinners (Warfarin/coumadin, for example), are particularly affected when cannabis is on board, so much so that the mixture can become toxic. Because of this mechanism, be cautious about introducing many different medicines or forms of cannabis into the body at the same time. If you're taking multiple medications and adding cannabinoids, do so in small increments and with patience. Be attentive to any changes in how you feel that may be linked to the interaction between your medication and cannabis, and not merely because of each component. The highest rates of success with cannabis use, in the long view, are when it is combined with multiple different types of other treatments or therapies (both within cannabis as a therapeutic and with respect to more traditional medical therapies). Attacking a single problem from different angles is more likely to meet success.

In many cases, traditional pharmaceuticals are a safe, tried-and-true option for achieving concrete goals. Nonetheless, there are occasions when pharmaceuticals simply aren't effective or have intolerable risks and side effects. Even for those who dislike their medication regimens, cannabis should not replace all of your medicines quickly or reflexively. Instead, I suggest that you first develop a comfort with cannabis along with your existing medications. Once you're comfortable and know how to adjust cannabis to achieve different means, then work with your healthcare provider to see if you can reduce some of your other medicines and fill in the gaps with cannabis. Don't discard medications on your own: there still might be subtle benefits that you are not aware of, which is why you should always discuss your medications with your healthcare provider. Even if the medicine might make you feel bad, it might be doing lifesaving work or have long-term importance you may not be considering.

Most importantly, if you have a serious medical condition or are already following a medication regimen, discuss potential cannabis interactions beforehand with a medical expert. Cannabis has direct effects on heart muscle, rhythm, and blood pressure. People who are on sensitive heart medicines must be aware of that, and their cardiologists should be aware that they are taking cannabis. In fact, discuss with all of your providers that you are going to be adding cannabis to your regimen. As a culture, we should be honest if we really want to do better. Patients who are intrigued or interested about cannabis deserve to be heard, and clinicians operating on incomplete information will give advice that is incomplete, if not potentially dangerous. There's no longer a reason to hide: the days when people were judged negatively for their cannabis use are dwindling. Today, even healthcare providers who are anti-cannabis are facing the unflinching reality that their patients are consuming cannabis just the same, and most would rather know about it so that they can better manage their patients accordingly. Ask if your provider is comfortable with their knowledge about cannabis. If they're not, give them this book.

Be Informed About Your Current Health Status

I tell my patients to have a complete physical before they start their cannabis journey. It's beneficial to know if you have health issues before you start any new medication treatment or healthcare routine. I have found that it's very common for otherwise knowledgeable people to be completely oblivious to major health concerns that are affecting them. For instance, some people with back pain may have serious bone issues; some people with skin conditions may have autoimmune disorders; some people with poor temperature regulation may have hormonal dysfunctions. And then there are the "silent diseases" like diabetes, heart disease, and certain cancers. As you'll learn in the chapters ahead, cannabis will impact many of these health concerns, so understanding your starting point can empower you to appreciate its true impact.

We also know that cannabis can dramatically alter the balance of infectious agents: the virus, bacteria, and fungus that lives within each of us in what is referred to as the *microbiome*.[3] Many people have underlying imbalances within their microbiome, which may or may not cause symptoms, such as digestive issues, bad breath, skin irritations, allergies, discomfort, and anxiety. These can all be signs of an underlying infection, even though they don't occur with typical symptoms like fever, chills, sweats, fatigue, and rashes. For some people, these concerns are part of their normal daily life.

Cannabis can influence these microbiome imbalances, and you may feel the effects as these infections are treated. For some, this change will bring welcome relief; for others the change can be jarring. This is why it's useful to know as much about your health as you can before starting a treatment that will modify your overall health status.

One Product May Really Do It All

The current medical model in the US relies on FDA approval for pharmaceuticals with very focused action on only one physiologic function at a time. This means that as we get older and our bodily functions diminish, we are almost by the nature of the health system pushed toward *polypharmacy*, or multiple pills for multiple ills, rather than away from it.

Cannabis medicine is completely different. It is inherently a multi-system actor, and it has shown itself to be a powerful agent in the other direction, helping to significantly reduce the need for a myriad of pharmaceuticals. This is another important reason to bring this book to your healthcare provider, so that when you bring cannabis into the mix, you can create a health plan that may include tapering off, or at least recalibrating, your existing medicinal dosages.

Evaluate Other Therapies

Let all of your therapeutic providers know that you are using cannabis as medicine, including mental health/behavioral therapists, physical therapy, occupational therapy, and so on. Most of the time, cannabis makes other therapies more effective, as it allows you to feel relaxed and present, and facilitates communication between different parts of the brain that allow therapy to work better. For instance, one goal of psychological therapy is for someone to gain awareness about subconscious desires, or how to handle life under duress or beyond their immediate awareness. Cannabis actually makes those connections easier.

The same is true for physical therapy. People who require physical therapy often find that the analgesic effects of cannabis help them during their sessions, allowing them to achieve better maneuverability so that they can strengthen and support the musculature around areas of pain and damage. So it not only adjusts the sensitivity of pain in the tissues, but it also increases blood flow and relaxes neighboring areas, allowing for greater flexibility.

With occupational therapies, if you are recovering from a stroke and relearning how to use utensils, cannabis is helpful for keeping you calm as you're remastering skills. A normal place of pain is an obstacle to effective therapy and learning. Easing that discomfort makes us more receptive to learning and change. That being said, THC versions of cannabis do have memory-impairing elements, which can add an obstacle to some aspects of the learning process.

Know Before You Go

Here are a few "rules of the road" so that you can begin your cannabis journey safely:

+ Don't consume intoxicating medicine and drive. In every state, impaired driving is illegal driving—and life-threatening. Operating a vehicle of any kind while consuming cannabis is potentially dangerous, no matter what your tolerance or comfort level. The effects of cannabis can affect your perception of time and distance, reaction time, focus, concentration, and interpretation of context. Driving under the influence of any drug is illegal, and it's as deadly and dangerous as driving drunk.

+ If you operate machinery while impaired by any medication or drug, even if they are legal, you can be arrested for DUI, face jail time and fines, and may injure yourself or others. While it seems true that more experienced cannabis consumers tend to be less distracted than those who are new to the experience of cannabis, the risk is not worth the odds; wait at least six hours after cannabis use before operating any equipment.

+ Don't take if pregnant or breastfeeding. Cannabis can cross the placental safety barriers and enter the mother's milk. Cannabis taken at smaller doses and/or at later stages of a pregnancy appears less likely to impact the fetus, but there are measurable effects in both circumstances that are still insufficiently understood. In time, it seems likely that some forms of cannabis may be compatible with pregnancy and/or breastfeeding, but until we know that potential benefits clearly outweigh the risks, the purest plan is to avoid cannabis.

+ Many people are anxious about having a medical procedure. Using cannabis before a procedure may be a helpful way to relax, but please let your doctor know about your consumption. Cannabis can interact with anesthesia, and you may require more sedation if you have cannabis in your system. While this may seem counterintuitive, a body accustomed to relief with cannabis may require additional medicine for optimal sedation.

+ Know who you are and what you need and want from cannabis. Having defined health goals can drastically improve your ability to make the right choices between different cannabis therapies so that you can achieve the results you are looking for.

+ Know what you cannot have from cannabis. Cannabis does not provide a quick fix with lasting results. It requires ongoing fine-tuning to develop a personally effective therapy for the long run. Your dosages will change if you develop tolerances, if product availability is inconsistent, or when your environment changes.

+ Know who you would enjoy consuming with (and/or alone). As you learned in this chapter, a positive cannabis experience is inextricable from the environment in which it is consumed. Efforts to create a supportive environment and community around the product are as important as the selection of consumables. Consider who you share your cannabis treatment outcomes with. Some adults are open with their friends and their own children, and some prefer to keep their cannabis use private. My experience is that different social dynamics warrant different approaches; a rebellious child may be more likely to avoid products their parents use, while a child who models their parents' behavior may be more curious and apt to follow suit. My impression is that honesty and clarity seem to cause the least amount of harm to everyone, and they promote an atmosphere of openness that is beneficial to your set and setting.

+ Store your products safely. If you have children, especially teenagers, in the house, keep your products in a temperature-stable, locked container. Luggage locks, home safes, and out-of-reach regions are preferable over storing them in a sock drawer or on a high shelf. The dosages recommended in this book are not intended for children, and children will often consume more than they should, especially when there is access to candy formulations. If a child consumes any unintended cannabis product, administer as much CBD or CBDA product as possible, and go directly to the emergency room of your local hospital.

+ Know your legal rights. Cannabis laws vary widely. There are national, state, and regional regulations that may limit the amount, type, and environments where cannabis can be purchased, grown, traded, given, or consumed. Working in federal buildings, traveling by air, and crossing state lines are unique situations where cannabis laws may differ from your expectations. Be aware of current laws and the risks of breaking them.

A Note About Cannabis Research

I've listed over one hundred scientific papers in this book so that you can see for yourself how much data exists, and that cannabis medicine is real science. Although the plant is very old, the science that surrounds it is still quite new. As you do your own research, you may find often confusing and contradictory findings. This doesn't bother me: in fact, it makes sense given the legal realities and challenges of studying cannabis without the ability to take a complete clinical picture into account.

Another reason why there is so much confusion about what cannabis does or does not do is because much of the research incorrectly assumes that it is all one unified substance. But as you've learned, the precise opposite is true. Within the natural variety of cannabis plants, and within any one plant itself, there can be an assortment of cannabinoid components, some opposing the actions of others. For instance, some cannabis compounds help to strengthen effective communication between cells, while others block clear channels of connection.

To this already complex scenario, add a wide variety of different methods of consuming cannabis, some of which contain significant amounts of heat (smoking/vaping) that can cause mutations and conversions of these same compounds, resulting in different effects. Adding further layers of complexity, much of the study of THC cannabinoids is based on the chemical analyses of isolated compounds in petri dishes, or the effects of cannabis on animals, not humans.

With so much variability, you can see that there is a daunting task ahead, as you attempt to reach a level of consistency and predictability with your treatments. The current paradigm of medical care—one pill for one ill—is not how cannabis medicine operates. With my guidance, you will be able to experiment and decide which products work best, and how and when to take them. Don't worry: within the cornucopia of molecules within cannabis, and the many formulations, there is a potential match to meet your needs. Through years of experience with thousands of patients who had previously failed with cannabis therapies, I have chaperoned their path to success.

What's Next

You're now ready to start investigating cannabis treatment protocols. The follow-ing chapters highlight the major areas where we know that cannabis can help, starting with mental health. Feel free to skip to the section where your greatest issues lie. However, I recommend that you read through the entire book. You'll be able to quickly see how synergistic cannabis therapies can be: they can affect your health at many levels at once. I also know that good health begets good health, so when you make the right changes to improve one area of your health, you may just find that you adopt better habits across the board. While each chapter provides a different lens from which you'll understand how cannabis interacts with different body systems, by reading through the entirety you can pick up on the nuances of how this therapy works overall.

All of the following recommendations are based on my experience treating thousands of patients with a wide variety of symptoms and conditions. They are also informed by the best scientific research available. However, it's important to understand that on many levels the scientific data is incomplete. It has been influ-enced by years of system-wide bias against cannabis in the scientific community. There still exists a certain level of social and political stigmatization. And because wild-type cannabis is still considered to be a Schedule I substance, there is very limited high-quality medical research. There are also almost no clinical studies based on illnesses that follow people over time, learning about long-term effects. Instead, we have lots of studies using CBD-dominant products, and a massive amount of THC-dominant animal and basic science studies.

Yet I don't see these limitations as insurmountable. I'm looking at all of this data through an informed lens. While it is logical to make recommendations for CBD products based on the scientific data we do have, my medical experience and the lessons I've learned from my patients by treating them over the course of their illnesses help me form appropriate recommendations that cover the full breadth and variety of cannabis products available. We do know that CBD and THC molecules are almost physically identical, hit many of the same receptors in the body, and produce comparable results (although sometimes they produce the opposite: remember set and setting!). We also know that the marketplace is ever-changing, producing many more types of products than any one study could consider. My goal for you is to find real solutions to your health problems with a fuller understanding of why cannabis may very well be a realistic and viable therapy for you.

PART TWO

Clinical Uses

CHAPTER 6

Mental Health Issues

While we might think about our feelings, moods, and emotions as intangible and impermanent states of mind, addressing concerns surrounding them turns out to be a solvable and tangible endeavor. Our emotional life, including the highs and the lows, is governed by cascades of chemistry that communicate messages from one brain region to the next. Like flowing water that carves deep channels in the ground, over time these chemical signals create strong, committed patterns of thought and emotion. For instance, your emotional response to crisis may always look like increased attention and anxiety, or, if you're battling daily stressors, toward the end of the day, you may regularly embrace the opportunity for calmness and a desire to retreat into a place of security.

When your mental health is strong, you can operate through the world at your peak, and you're more resilient when facing daily stumbling blocks. But when your day-to-day life is hindered by an inability to control your thoughts or emotions, I know that it can be debilitating. However, you don't have to suffer—or take medications with intolerable side effects. I've found that while cannabis works best when paired with other medications, it can also work well as a singular tool for addressing a wide variety of mental health issues. I've seen people with crippling PTSD, incapacitating anxiety, intense depression, and frustrating ADHD effectively address these issues and resume their lives. For some, the change is rapid and dramatic.

Truth vs. Fiction

Contrary to the drug abuse resistance campaigns that spread prejudicial, biased, and misinformed concepts from the 1930s through the 1990s, excessive cannabis use does not lead to apathy and psychosis. Paid television, radio, and print campaigns lied to the public: movies showed cannabis smokers losing their minds, jumping out of windows, or embarking on a life of crime. We were erroneously led to believe that using cannabis would somehow strip us of an otherwise healthy interest in daily life.

We do know that everyone's experience, even with the same cannabis products, often yields dramatically different results. As you've learned, every aspect of your environment surrounding your use will also affect outcomes, so what works one day may not be the exact same prescription necessary for the next. When it comes to mental health, the volume of use is an important variable to making sure that your experience is pleasant and effective. Small doses that at first only barely feel effective rarely lead to long-lasting psychological discomfort. At higher doses or increased frequency, you may experience disorientation, confusion, panic, paranoia, extreme depression, or anxiety. These symptoms will go away with time, fluids, and sleep.

The key to resolving your mental health complaints will be finding the "just right" dose for you. This is why I always say, *go low and slow*. Within a few weeks, you will be able to recognize when you are feeling better and when you've had too much.

How Cannabis Affects the Brain

Cannabis affects the brain in a number of different ways. The endocannabinoid system itself acts as a regulatory system for emotional responses. Studies have shown that one of its key functions may be to ensure that an appropriate response is mounted during incidences of pain, learning, and emotional/psychological stressors.[1] An elevated level of endocannabinoids, either produced in the body or coming from cannabis, has a calming effect.[2] We know this because there are people who are born with endocannabinoid deficiency. The repercussion can look like anxiety, depression, or a predilection to PTSD or pain. In contrast, individuals flush with cannabinoids tend to be happy, satisfied, and free of pain and depression.

Cannabinoids allow the brain to change the path of well-worn thought channels, hacking our emotional and cognitive rigidity so that new ideas and feelings can emerge. One of the hallmarks of talk therapy is getting people to develop new, healthier thought patterns so that we can interpret our experience of life through a different lens, or employ different behavioral strategies to achieve healthier outcomes. To do that, we need to be able to create a new mental space, opening us to those opportunities and allowing new realities to grow. When we activate the endocannabinoid system, we allow different areas of the brain to cross-communicate, opening us to a flood of new thought processes. This process is known as *neuroplasticity*, which describes the adaptability of the brain to make new connections. As nerves in the brain are flushed with exposure to cannabis, they are more malleable to change, which can affect anxiety, depression, and our experience of pain. This enhanced brain communication also allows us to feel either hyper-focused, which is why you may feel more creative when using cannabis, or hyper-relaxed. To some, focused creativity looks more like distraction. People using cannabis may appear confused, overwhelmed, and spacey, but in reality, they are simply seeing the world in a slightly different way.

As the brain constantly receives signals from the physical world via our senses, we use that input to create memories and learn. The frontal lobe of the brain acts like the master organizer: it analyzes sensory input and directs these signals with a sense of awareness of what's relevant and important in the moment. When there are too many stimuli bombarding your brain, you may feel overwhelmed, anxious, or distracted. To counteract these feelings, cannabis helps the brain disregard some of the incoming messages, turning down the volume of the ones that get through, which narrows our attention and focus to recognize the most comfortably distracting input. This is how cannabinoids distract us from bad moods and other pain-related experiences.

Endocannabinoids may play a protective role by reducing inflammation.[3] Some of the symptoms of poor mental health include feeling tension and pain in your body; we also know that those in chronic pain are often depressed. Studies show that when people take traditional anti-inflammatories, like ibuprofen (Advil), there is a positive impact on emotional health and mental health.[4] Cannabis is known to act as a strong anti-inflammatory, acting on both the brain and the body to relieve pain and improve mood.

What's more, cannabinoid and terpenoid compounds serve as powerful buffers against the detrimental effects of persistent stress, which is mediated by our natural stress hormone system (the cortisol and adrenaline released during a fight/flight/freeze response). The presence of cannabinoid molecules disrupts each part of the response so that fewer stress hormones are released, and fewer bind to receptors, leading to a decrease in the long-term effects of these hormones. By doing so, cannabis is indirectly influencing emotion, mood, energy levels (fatigue or vigor), and memory.[5] For instance, we know that cannabis activates the heart and increases heart rate. When people using cannabis feel their heart racing, they are also experiencing a release of endorphins and stress hormones. As a result, they may interpret their heart racing as "scary." This experience commonly sets off feelings of paranoia—the presence of fear without attribution—that is associated with cannabis: the user is sensing a physical change in the body that makes them feel stressed or anxious. In reality, you are interpreting your reaction to cannabis on many different levels: you have a real physical manifestation, you have the interpretation of that physical manifestation, and you assign a different cause to that physical manifestation. This is why setting up a calm environment and trying to achieve a level of mindfulness is so critical for a positive cannabis therapy experience. Many of my patients report that listening to calming music and enjoying good food and good company helps make their therapy more effective.

Addressing Depression and Anxiety

Depression and anxiety are two of the most common reasons why people come to me for guided cannabis therapies. Cannabis does not cure either anxiety or depression, but it offers a distraction that allows you to focus on something else besides the feelings, thoughts, and cycles of negativity. At the same time that cannabinoids turn down the volume of negative stimuli, they flush the brain with neutral and positive signals, which reduces the intensity of maladaptive thought patterns. To my mind, and in the results I see with many of my patients, these two functions allow cannabis to replace the internal wiring/signaling of pain with one of joy.

As a medication, cannabis restores the brain's chemical equilibrium in ways similar to how antidepressants are designed to work. Antidepressants mimic brain chemicals or influence them. First, cannabis acts on the same systems of brain chemistry, making antidepressants more efficient. And like many depression, anxiety, and pain medications, cannabinoids stimulate neural growth so that the brain has stronger connectivity, enabling its natural chemical messengers to work more efficiently. In the future, we may discover that cannabis is in fact an effective treatment option on its own as it floods the brain with joy molecules, but as of this writing, it's not clear. We do know that in addition to improving neural communication, cannabis molecules act directly on the same receptors that bind to our naturally occurring chemistry of joy. The chemical structure of THC is similar to the brain chemical *anandamide*, which is our principal happiness molecule that activates and facilitates feelings of joy.[6] The same brain circuitry that responds to anandamide responds to THC.

Most depression and anxiety medications are used in a precise, system-specific manner, operating at a single receptor or chemical pathway; very few besides cannabis impact more than one region of the brain, or at the same time also impact regions of the body. Cannabis can also be used to address isolated components of depression and anxiety, including lethargy, fatigue, pain, aggressive or self-injurious behaviors, and others. Think about the interlocking gears of a clock and how they connect to keep the clock running. Some traditional anxiety and depression medicines may replace faulty gears with a better fitting gear, or they may help existing gears run more smoothly. Cannabis doesn't necessarily replace the gears themselves, but it extends their access in a way that still creates the desired effect. Cannabis also seems to smooth out areas of rust so that the clock continues to work well. In this way, cannabis both facilitates the interaction of all the gears to work synergistically (the whole brain) or works on just one gear.

One well-known problem with antidepressants is that the ramp-up time for these medications is very long: it can take up to six to eight weeks for anxiety and depression medications to start working. That is not the case for cannabis, where the ramp up can be as quick as two weeks to achieve a steady balance. For those suffering from acute anxiety or depression, that immediacy has tremendous value. Unlike traditional antidepressants, cannabis is not associated with weight gain, reduced sex drive, hormonal disruption (acne, mood swings), or sleep disturbances. In fact, it can improve all of these conditions, which you'll see throughout the book.

Some medications used to treat anxiety, like benzodiazepines—Xanax, Valium, Ativan—are not only dangerous and addictive; they're very short-acting. As satisfying as these quick-acting options are, the medications are rapidly habit forming and easily hit a level of tolerance, incurring a need for steadily increasing dose requirements. Despite the popular and misinformed rumor, cannabis is not any more addictive than caffeine. While I commonly see patients who use cannabis regularly for improving their mental health, rarely does it interfere with the rest of their daily lives.

Using cannabis as a therapy in the presence of a healthy environment enhances your ability to improve mood, and over time, your mood may become consistently more relaxed and positive. As my patients ramp up on cannabis, they can work with their doctors to lower the amount of other depression and anxiety prescription medications—or drop them entirely.

MEET SYLVIA

Sylvia was forty-five when we first met over a telehealth appointment. Even though she looked put together, I could see from the disarray of her home in the background that she really needed help. She told me that she had reached her limit: the unending demands on her time, including nonstop laundry, cooking healthy meals for her family, and trying to keep a livable clean home, made her feel like she was at her wit's end. Her teenage daughters were stressing her out, which was putting a strain on her marriage. Some days she had trouble getting motivated to get out of bed and deal with all of her responsibilities, and her constant worry kept her up at night. She had tried antidepressants and spoke to a therapist earlier that year, but she was unhappy with the weight she had gained and how the medicine affected her libido, which was one of the few joys of married life. She knew she was drinking wine to relax her enough to get to sleep, but it wasn't a great strategy: she was gaining weight, and on the nights she drank, she would wake up when the sugar crashed and wouldn't be able to get back to sleep because of ruminating thoughts and a recurring need to visit the bathroom. She was ready to try something new to help her get through the day without feeling like she was dragging the whole family down.

I asked Sylvia if she had ever tried cannabis in the past, and she told me she had back in college, but didn't have a great experience. I reassured her that we would be able to work together to find a combination of products that would help ease her mind without affecting her thinking. Because she lived in Massachusetts, she would be able to get a medical cannabis card, which meant that she had a plethora of options available. For daytime use to ease her anxiety, I suggested she start with a low-dose CBD chocolate, which would be non-intoxicating, relaxing, calming, and long-lasting. At the end of the day, she could try a CBD:THC tincture that was shorter acting, which would bring immediate relief so that she could unwind without turning to alcohol. When she was getting ready for bed, she could take a THC tablet, which would help keep her asleep for a solid six- to eight-hour stretch.

About a month later we had a follow-up appointment. Sylvia looked rested and comfortable. She let me know that the chocolates had been successful, and within a few weeks she was able to find the right dose of tincture to help her unwind at the end of the day without a glass or two of wine. She wasn't taking all of my recommendations every day, using them only when needed, and overall felt like she was more in control. She seemed to be feeling better about her relationship with her daughters and her husband, and had more energy and felt less frazzled during the day.

I was really pleased with her results and explained that I wasn't surprised that she didn't need the cannabis products as much, because they had helped rewire her sleep patterns, which rejuvenated her energy and thinking. Going forward, she could focus on the positive aspects of her day, and when she did feel blue or started to worry, she had convenient, adaptable tools to address her anxious mind, without any additional concerns to manage.

Treating Eating Disorders

We don't fully understand if eating disorders are governed partially or completely by the endocannabinoid system. There is a clear connection between addressing the symptoms of appetite, anxiety, depression, and obsessive thinking with cannabis, yet the precise tangle of interaction between these disparate systems has not been fully investigated. Because they often share similar features with those suffering from obsessive, ruminative, and anxiety and/or depression disorders, patients struggling with eating disorders like anorexia and bulimia are typically treated with antidepressants. Psychiatric literature supports this pharmaceutical approach to therapy, and many people attest to experiencing some improvement. However, my patients with eating disorders have more lasting success with cannabis therapies than they generally have with traditional antidepressants alone. It is helping people manage their appetite, address symptoms of anxiety and/or depression, and navigate their impulses surrounding food.

Treating Obsessive-Compulsive Disorder and Post-traumatic Stress Disorder

Obsessive-compulsive disorder and post-traumatic stress disorder are two mental health issues that combine unending suffering and rumination: it's like memory gone haywire. The brain is basically a network of neurons, and when a certain channel of neurons is firing too strongly or too often, the brain is supposed to redirect or move away from that signal. Ruminating thoughts occur when the brain cannot redirect, and it results in overactive nerve channels. Cannabis lowers the volume on the expression of those hyperactive nerves, inhibiting their message. By providing a mental space to stop the cycle of fixation, sufferers can first increase the amount of time between unpleasant thoughts, and gradually fill that time with productive alternatives, instead of recollecting painful memories and reliving past trauma.

Traditional medicines do not soften short-term memory in the same way that cannabis can. They are often difficult to dose, they must accompany regular and expert medical guidance and oversight, and they often don't have lasting benefit, which leaves sufferers frustrated. At too high a dose, they are so powerful that they don't allow the one suffering to develop his or her own new strategies to replace the persistent conveyor belt of traumatic memories. Or, the medications are not powerful enough to stop the unending thoughts.

Cannabis therapies may be a better alternative to treating OCD and PTSD because on top of a foundation of improved calmness, comfort, and a small degree of joy that cannabis provides, cannabis strongly affects short-term memory, offering a much-needed vacation from rumination. Cannabis frees someone with obsessive thinking so that they can redirect their own thoughts and channel their thinking more productively.

MEET STEVE

At thirty-one, Steve was the prototypical tech overachiever. However, he knew that his compulsive behavior was probably the reason he was consistently passed over for a promotion. During the day, he was in the habit of slowly double-checking his work, and at night, when he should be resting, he was up late worrying whether he had offended anyone in the office. He was doing better on his OCD medications, but he wasn't achieving all the results he wanted.

When I met with him, we discussed his previous experience with cannabis. He told me he smoked a lot of pot in high school and college and that it did relax him, but he hadn't thought of it as anything more than a social lubricant. He explained that he didn't want to feel intoxicated during work hours and certainly couldn't afford to be less productive. I suggested that he try a high-CBD, low-THC product, delivered as dissolving tablets, which he could easily "microdose" throughout the day, placing the tablets under his tongue. I explained that this regimen was considered a high dose, but it would offer him quick relief and work well with his existing medications, without any distracting effects or loss of work productivity. In time, he would be able to drop down to fewer doses over the course of the day to maintain the same level of calm.

To my surprise, Steve continues to use the same high dose I started him on, and he is always pleased to tell me that he is just as productive as always. He reports that nothing has worked as well as cannabis to treat his OCD.

You Don't Have to Go Through Life Stressed

We all have stressors in our lives, and sometimes they bubble up beyond our control. No matter the source of stress, it is healthy and important to find ways to resolve the source of problems and restore an even-tempered equilibrium. For some, a walk does the trick. For others, it's meditation or yoga. For a growing number of people, cannabis has become an effective tool for stress relief.

Stress can range from subtle mood changes, lasting aggravation, and at the other end of the spectrum, symptoms of dissociation where you lose touch with what you are doing or even where you are. I remember one patient who called me in the middle of a panic attack, not knowing where she was and feeling completely out of control. I walked her through a few behavioral techniques to calm down on the spot, but her mind was spinning. I then recommended that she take a puff on her vape pen, which she had forgotten was in her purse. Within twenty-five seconds she reported that her symptoms were plateauing and coming within a range where she felt in control. I was glad she was able to locate the pen, because I know that no other medication she could have possibly taken would have worked as fast.

For some, cannabis is the physical manifestation of meditation. Cannabis easily distracts us from our unwanted thoughts. It can relax the mind as powerfully as it can soothe the body. It can allow you to take a step back and relax. You can even incorporate your dosing into a meditation practice.

Treating Adult Attention Deficit Hyperactivity Disorder (ADD/ADHD)

Another component of mental health is the ability to place the right amount of attention to a specific task, as well as the interpretation and memory of that attention. ADD/ADHD presents differently for different people, and although it's often spoken about in the context of children, many adults suffer from it. Some are fidgety and have difficulty attending to anything. Others have hyper-focus and cannot let go of a certain task. Still others can focus appropriately, but can't remember what they were attending to because they are plagued with competing thoughts and distractions.

Cannabis temporarily curtails some streams of short-term memory so that users can stay in the moment, unburdened by emotional or sensory intrusions, and complete the task at hand. In many ways it quiets an overactive brain. Compared to traditional ADD/ADHD medications like Adderall, Ritalin, guanfacine, and others, cannabis is equally stimulating without leading to a loss of appetite, insomnia, and persistent heart racing. It can bring relaxation to both a hyper-focused and strongly divided mind, and can ease the stressful burden of ruminative self-assessment that often comes with ADD.

Because symptoms of ADD are not so far off from typical stressors, many people with this disorder have been "self-medicating" with cannabis without ever getting a formal diagnosis. So it's no surprise that this strategy works. However, we live in a culture that has stigmatized self-medicating to the point that it is a pejorative term. It suggests that someone is relying excessively on, or abusing, drugs or alcohol to make it through the day. In my experience, it is clear that cannabis does help address these conditions, and even without a formal diagnosis or an authoritative awareness of their condition, this strategy is actually a form of valuable self-care.

MEET LESLIE

My patient Leslie, who at age seventy had ADHD and was a longtime user of cannabis, was able to transition to a more effective guided cannabis approach. Leslie is an amateur artist who could never seem to commit to one medium of art over another. As quickly as she found herself drawn to one form of expression, she would find herself drawn to another and another. With support, Leslie found that CBD-dominant products helped her relax her wandering mind enough to complete works in progress, and THC-dominant products that she used from time to time could launch her creativity in energetic spurts. As the years went on, she discovered mixtures and regimens of cannabis that she could turn on or turn up to enable more useful control over her inattentive tendencies.

Sample Regimens for Treating Mental Health Concerns

Our endocannabinoid system can be modified to create what I call a better *tone*, a mental baseline of relaxed attention. Cannabinoids can help us regulate emotions and cognition to achieve a balanced, manageable daily experience. No matter the short-term timing of medicine administration, there are long-term benefits for the sustained use of cannabis, particularly for treating mental health issues. My patients who have been using cannabis consistently report fewer mood swings, more consistent comfort, less depression, less anxiety, better sleep, and better quality of life. Others use cannabis on a more sporadic basis for a brief vacation from mounting stressors. Still others use intermittently, perhaps a week on followed by a week off; these patients often develop less tolerance and can sustain lower dosages for longer periods of time.

While everyone will have a slightly different experience, I have found that the following suggestions offer the most relief for the mental health issues discussed in this chapter.

+ **Onset timing:** The speed of onset will be your personal choice.

+ **Short-acting versus longer-lasting:** Short-acting options provide quick relief from an excessive mental burden, while long-lasting options provide a foundation of support for a challenging day. As you become more comfortable with the effects of cannabis, you can switch to a microdosing strategy, increasing dosages to provide stronger relief.

+ **Daytime or nighttime:** New users should explore nighttime consumption, which will avoid any uncomfortable impact on daily experience and help you sleep while you are becoming accustomed to the effects of cannabinoids.

+ **Euphoric/non-euphoric:** For most people, CBD options will keep them balanced during the day without affecting their productivity. In rare exceptions, THC, rather than CBD, helps people think more clearly. For these people, THC may not cause distraction or euphoria during the day, and it may actually help them to better function at a "normal" acceptable baseline. If you suffer from depression, you may benefit from THC products. If you are more anxious, you may benefit from more CBD.

+ **Compare products:** Compare the products containing specific terpenes and flavonoids to the master list in chapter one to make sure you are getting the benefits you are looking for. I believe that terpenes and flavonoids may offer more nuanced control of mental health issues, but this has not yet been fully explored in rigorous scientific studies.

+ **Product recommendation—lotions:** Believe it or not, lotions that are liberally applied to the face, and even the body, can address mental health concerns. The muscle relaxation effects of cannabinoids are dramatic, and just as a good massage might relieve daily stressors, so, too, can cannabis topicals. For instance, many of my athletic patients use cannabis topicals as a part of their daily regimen to address stress and pain. Topicals also offer a way to get a low dose of THC throughout the day without the distracting cognitive effects.

+ **Cannabis and medications:** Adding cannabis products to your existing prescription regimen will make mental health medications work better. Do not stop taking prescription medications without fully consulting your prescribing healthcare provider. You should feel comfortable with cannabis and how it might make you feel before you entertain reducing other medicines or getting off them.

Don't Hesitate to See a Therapist

Even with cannabis on board, some people will benefit from having a professional guide them through a healthier understanding of their reality, including an accurate interpretation of their thought processes and behaviors.

Today's mental health providers are more open-minded to cannabis as a therapeutic adjunct. Talk about it with your therapist and see if they have suggestions on how best to incorporate it with your talk therapy. My data shows that patients who use cannabis during their therapy find that the process is easier: you may find that you are more amenable to healthy redirection.

Lastly, consider tapping into the joy you can derive from other healthy habits, and make those experiences part of your daily life. I often tell my patients that even small and seemingly insignificant successes make us feel good, distract us from negative thoughts, and bolster self-esteem. Walks around the block, eating nutritious and tasty foods, enjoyable television, spending time in nature, listening to beautiful music, and experiencing beautiful artwork can all enhance our existing endocannabinoid system. The more we can augment our natural endocannabinoid baseline, the better we will feel about ourselves.

CHAPTER 7

Sleep Disturbances

Almost everyone struggles with getting a good night's rest from time to time. Many also face sleeplessness every night. Either scenario can be problematic: besides feeling overtired and restless, insomnia can cause debilitating health issues that often lead to a circular effect—any disease caused by poor sleep can keep the cycle of poor sleep going. The same is true for mental health: inconsistent sleep patterns can cause us to feel out of control, anxious, and depressed, ultimately creating a cycle of discomfort. What's more, poor sleep leads to making poor choices in terms of food and exercise routines, and it's directly associated with obesity, diabetes, and other chronic conditions.[1]

The conventional way we treat sleep issues has its own host of problems. Many traditional medicines that address sleep issues are addictive and have serious side effects. Even over-the-counter agents like antihistamines, NyQuil, or supplements like melatonin do not always work or come with unsustainable side effects. Or you may be treating your sleep issue with the wrong medication for your particular problem.

Let's look at the most popular traditional sleep medications:

+ Benzodiazepines and so-called *hypnotics* are anti-anxiety medications that are frequently used to promote relaxation and sleep. The most popular are

Ambien, Ativan, Librium, Valium, Xanax, Lunesta, and Sonata. The problem with these medications is that you're only supposed to take them for six weeks, but people stay on them forever. Long-term use often requires the user to increase the dosage as tolerance develops, and that tolerance is potentially lethal. One interesting study appearing in the *British Medical Journal* showed that death from all causes tripled when people stay on benzodiazepines for extended periods of time.[2] Even in the short term, some people taking these medications complain of a "hangover effect," meaning that they continue to feel groggy the following day. Many of my patients taking these medications have reported bizarre behaviors, including sleepwalking, nighttime eating while asleep, and even driving while asleep.

+ Dual orexin receptor antagonists are a new class of medications that include Dayvigo, Belsomra, and daridorexant. These medications suppress the wake drive so that you fall asleep quickly and stay asleep. This class is typically more expensive than other prescription sleep medications and can also cause daytime drowsiness.

+ Doxylamine, diphenhydramine, chlorphenamine, cinnarizine, hydroxyzine, and promethazine are antihistamines found in the over-the-counter medications that include Benadryl, NyQuil, and Tylenol PM. Low-dose doxepin is a tricyclic antidepressant but has similar antihistamine activity. These medications are often taken either before bed to help make you sleepy or in the middle of the night to knock you out if you wake up. They work by blocking the histamine receptors in the brain and spinal cord, causing drowsiness. While these medications do not require a prescription, it doesn't mean that they do not have side effects. In fact, many complain of dizziness, disturbed coordination, constipation, dry mouth, difficulty urinating, upset stomach, blurred vision, tremor, loss of appetite, headache, or nausea. The histamine system affects many different fundamental operating networks throughout the body, which is why these medicines have a wide array of potentially uncomfortable side effects.

+ Melatonin is sold as a supplement in the US, but in many other countries it requires a prescription. Many people take melatonin because they think it's a harmless, natural alternative, but this isn't really the case. Melatonin is helpful in getting you to sleep, but it can also cause mild side effects including nausea, dizziness, and headaches. And as a natural hormone, melatonin can impact other body systems.

+ Antidepressants have modest sleep-enhancing effects, but other than doxepin, they aren't recommended for routine use because the sedating effects tend to be short-lived, and this category of medication can come with significant side effects. In addition to some temporary sedative effects, these medications increase serotonin and norepinephrine in the brain and sometimes effectively address underlying mood states that may be contributing to insomnia. Other antidepressant medications, including trazodone, Remeron, and amitriptyline, are the most common off-label ones prescribed for insomnia.

+ Dietary supplements are sometimes marketed for improving sleep, but very few show reproduceable benefits through formal scientific analysis. Examples include chamomile, kava, L-theanine, lavender, magnesium, nightshade, tryptophan, valerian, hops, and glycine.

Common Causes of Chronic Insomnia

The causes for interruption of sleep are multidimensional, and can include mental health issues, physical discomfort, and pain. If you suffer from any of the following, it may be contributing to your sleep problems:

Psychiatric conditions:
Anxiety
Depression
Post-traumatic stress disorder
Substance abuse

Medical conditions:
Arthritis
Asthma

Brain tumors

Cancer

Chronic fatigue syndrome

Chronic obstructive pulmonary disease

Dermatologic (e.g., pruritus, fungal or bacterial skin infections)

Diabetes

Fibromyalgia

Gastroesophageal reflux

Headache

Heart failure

History of strokes

Human immunodeficiency virus (HIV)

Hypertension

Hyperthyroidism

Ischemic heart disease

Lyme disease

Menopause

Neurodegenerative diseases (e.g., Alzheimer's disease, dementia, Parkinson's disease)

Neuromuscular disorders

Pain

Pregnancy

Traumatic brain injury

Urinary nocturia

Medications:

Alcohol

Antidepressants

Beta antagonists

Bronchodilators

Caffeine

Central nervous system depressants

Central nervous system stimulants

Diuretics

Glucocorticoids

Other Sleep Disorders:

Circadian rhythm disorders

Delayed sleep-wake phase disorder

Irregular sleep-wake rhythm disorder

Restless leg syndrome

Shift work disorder

Sleep apnea

The Caplan Sleep Quality Questionnaire

How is your life impacted by your sleeplessness? Are your activities limited? Your mood changed? Poor sleep affects your life more than just being late for work or feeling tired all day. It can impact your physical and mental health, thwart social relationships, and ultimately even shorten your life. Understanding your own sleep challenges and how they are affecting your life right now is the first step to identifying the types of cannabis products that might help. Remember, the guided cannabis approach takes into account not only finding a product that works, but understanding your needs and your environment, and how that product interacts with both. The best match will take into account all three legs of the stool—your needs, your environment, and the appropriate product—and can accommodate changes in each as they arise.

1. On a scale from 1–10, how would you rate the quality of your sleep over the past week? <4 = bad; >7 = good
2. How many days each week do you have a good night of sleep? <3 = bad; >5 = good
3. About how many hours, out of twenty-four total, are you typically sound asleep (not just in bed)? Be sure to include naps, if any. <5 = bad; >7 = good

If your total for questions 1–3 is 13 or less, you have a serious sleep problem; between 13–20 you have suboptimal sleep that can be improved. If your total is 20 or greater, you are having a good week of sleep.

4. Do you have trouble getting to sleep or staying asleep?
    a. Getting to sleep
    b. Staying asleep
    c. Both

5. When you have trouble staying asleep, when do you typically awaken and have trouble getting back to sleep?
    a. Soon after falling asleep
    b. Middle of the night
    c. Early in the morning
    d. Just prior to when I normally wake up

Question 4 highlights what type of sleep disturbance you may have. Question 5 will help you determine the type of product to take upon awakening in the middle of the night to satisfy your sleep needs without next-day grogginess.

6. Is your sleep often interrupted by outside forces (noises, movements) or bodily sensations (pain, itching, the bathroom, etc.)?

7. When you are in bed, not sleeping, are you ruminating about daytime concerns (work, family, other stresses)?

8. Do you have a diagnosed sleep disorder or medical condition that's impacting your sleep (see sidebar)?

9. Do you sleep with the lights on, even small lights coming from electronics? Do you watch TV or have your phone nearby while in bed?

10. Is your bedtime routine inconsistent?

Questions 6–10 highlight aspects of sleep hygiene that may pose opportunities for improvement. If you answer yes to any of these questions, see recommendations later in the chapter to address these environmental changes.

11. Are you hoping to replace any current medications with cannabis?

12. Are you planning to use any medications concurrently with cannabis to help you sleep better?

13. Are you open to intoxication during the evening?
14. Do you have any responsibilities that you need to be potentially available for during the night (young children, etc.)?

These last questions will help guide you to making the right choice within the framework of existing cannabis products.

Cannabis Offers a Variety of Antidotes to Sleep Issues

Treating sleep issues with cannabis is universally successful: it is one of the best, safest sleep aids we have. Thousands of my patients have reported that they feel well-slept, more energized, and often more productive after they've used a cannabis product at nighttime. Once the welcome sleep arrives, it is often deep, with less sleep disturbance, longer duration, and ultimately more restful. This fact alone might be the reason why cannabis seems to be effective for so many disparate illnesses: the effects of cannabis on ameliorating pain, stress, and chronic illness may all be related to its ability to enhance and effect sleep.

The impact that cannabis can have on your sleep concerns is influenced by factors such as dosage, ratio of cannabinoid ingredients, prior cannabis experience, timing, route of administration, and, of course, the quality of product being consumed. Cannabis products act in the exact same way that your inherent endocannabinoid system interacts with the different mechanisms that regulate sleep. First, it helps to regulate circadian rhythms. Second, it enhances REM sleep. Third, it increases the ability to achieve mental and physical calmness and relaxation, providing a distraction from the ruminating thoughts and pain that keep us up at night. Together, these mechanisms allow for a pendulum swing away from chaotic or disturbed sleep and toward establishing sleep habits that are more regular and effective.

Cannabis and Circadian Rhythms

Our internal organs, including those that regulate sleep, are supposed to operate in a synchronized fashion known as *a circadian rhythm*, which is linked to a twenty-four-hour day. Some sleep disorders are caused by a circadian rhythm disruption, which can occur from any number of sources, including hormonal changes, schedule impacts, external stimuli, and poor eating habits. For instance, it is very common for older, retired adults who have the freedom to stay up late at night reading or watching television to lose track of time, ending up with too few hours of sleep. The subtle, short-term disruptions do add up to meaningful health impacts. Over time, this disruption not only affects the quality of our sleep; it can affect many other aspects of our overall health, including weight gain, heart disease, and even diabetes.[3]

We also know that our circadian rhythm is intimately connected with our endocannabinoid system. Sleep is, in part, governed by a tiny gland in the brain that is thought of as the master clock. This gland is known to be impacted by the cannabinoids already in our endocannabinoid system as well as external cannabis products.[4] When our circadian rhythm is disrupted, cannabinoids can act as a reset to our circadian clock, and they do so by activating the brain's microglial cells. Some cannabinoids can also hack your rhythm to get you back on track by promoting relaxation, comfort, and reducing distracting signals. For instance, shift workers who work at night and have to sleep during the day use cannabis products to help them align their schedule with their desired sleep regimen.

Cannabis and the Stages of Sleep

Having a great night's sleep means that you have slept soundly through multiple cycles of quiet sleep and active sleep. Quiet sleep takes place in three stages: drowsiness, light sleep, and deep sleep. Light sleep is really the first phase of true sleep. Deep sleep occurs when the brain becomes less responsive to external stimuli, making it difficult to wake up. These three stages of quiet sleep alternate with periods of active sleep, which is referred to as *rapid eye movement (REM) sleep*. During this time, your body is still; your mind is racing and dreaming. We typically have between three to five cycles of quiet/REM sleep per night, occurring every 90 to 120 minutes. During active REM sleep, your muscles will contract, releasing stored cannabinoids into the bloodstream, naturally promoting better sleep.

A plentiful amount of cannabinoids is necessary for sleep. However, cannabinoid levels can be limited when there are also low levels of 2-Octyl γ-bromoacetoacetate, a natural brain enzyme present in our cerebrospinal fluid. When both are in high levels, cannabis is thought to enhance deep, REM sleep.[5] Because this is your active stage of sleep, you may find that dreams are more intense and memorable, and you may even feel more aware while sleeping.

The Balancing Quality of Cannabis

The presence of cannabinoids inherently makes us feel more comfortable as they balance hormone signaling and communication. This enhanced comfort is necessary for experiencing good sleep. Think about the body as a pool containing different colored fluids, and each color is meant to flow toward a specific destination and occasionally interact with other colors. Each color represents a hormone, which is a focused signal that allows one part of the body to communicate with another. When these signals are delivered in a healthy fashion, we feel comfortable and have greater access to joy. Yet when there is too much of any one hormone, or color, other colors cannot transmit their signals properly. The result is an imbalance, which is what we feel as pain, sadness, fatigue, anxiety, or illness.

Lasting deep sleep depends on having effective hormonal signaling channels. The endocannabinoid system helps to restore hormonal balance, which then facilitates optimal signaling. By supporting the endocannabinoid system with external cannabis, you are helping to bring the excessive colors back into their natural balance.

Considerations for a Good Night's Sleep

+ **Onset timing:** Fast-acting products are sedating. They will also promote healthy sleep by relaxing muscles, calming busy thoughts, and allowing you to focus on pleasant thoughts rather than ruminating on your worries of the day. To fall asleep rapidly, quick-acting options include a tincture under the tongue, dissolving sublingual tablet or strip, well-positioned topicals applied to select regions of the body (arms and shoulders, face, and thighs), or vaporizing/nebulizing inhaled cannabinoids. Higher dosages can speed up the process of getting to sleep, as well as affect duration. Too much can impede comfort and prevent sleep.

+ **Short-acting versus longer-lasting:** Treating insomnia takes into account the short-acting and long-lasting effects of specific cannabis products. Choosing among the quick-acting options described above will help you get to sleep, and can also be used upon wakening in the middle of the night without worrying that you would sleep through your morning routine. Choose longer-lasting options for help staying asleep. These include ingesting edibles or tinctures, topical patches, or slow-release pills. Some people who have difficulty getting to sleep and staying asleep do best with a combination of short-acting and long-lasting options taken at the same time: the long-lasting edible will begin working when the short-acting option is no longer effective.

  Unlike prescription medications that linger in the body for extended periods of time and create addiction, cannabis operates through short-lived signaling. This means that even long-lasting products only offer temporary relief, and they can be used repeatedly to create long-term solutions without necessarily causing addiction. The temporary action also means that cannabis is not as incapacitating as some prescription sleep aids.

+ **Daytime or nighttime:** The action of cannabinoids is inextricable from its set and setting. The same product that feels sedating at nighttime might feel pleasantly relaxing or offer focused attention during the day. Some of my patients report that when they use cannabis products during the day, they feel more energetic, and are then more tired at night and sleep better. It's quite common for people with sleep issues to be sedentary during the day, and using cannabis during the day can support improved levels of activity.

  There are some products, often using the terms *sedating/indica*, that are marketed as sedating no matter when they are consumed. In fact, the mixture of additional terpenes, flavonoids, and botanicals is what amplifies the calming qualities. For nighttime use, look for a soothing product containing high levels of THC and other CBD-derived cannabinoids, as well as beta-caryophyllene, linalool, and myrcene. You can also experiment with taking a long-lasting edible hours before sleep to observe its sedating effects and how they are influenced by a variety of different set and settings.

+ **Euphoric/non-euphoric:** A mix of cannabinoids is critical for ideal relief and avoidance of tolerance. Individual cannabinoids alone may work, but combinations work better. Most people who have used cannabis in the past gravitate toward THC products. For consumers who aren't used to THC, these products can be overwhelming at first, leaving them feeling too sedated or too stimulated, depending on their set and setting. For new consumers, I typically recommend a protocol that is either neutral or less THC-dominant, focusing on CBD products, or an even ratio of THC and CBD. Overall, both CBD and THC can normalize circadian rhythms, enhance REM sleep, and provide a more comfortable internal sleep environment. THC products are better for someone whose emotional state or overactive mind is keeping them up at night. For example, a PTSD army veteran might benefit from the calming features of THC so that he or she can feel less anxious, at peace, and temporarily distracted from the otherwise recurring disturbing emotions and interruptions of memory that keep her awake.

+ **Cannabis and medications:** Adding cannabis products to your existing sleep prescription regimen will make it work better. They are often chemically compatible and processed in the body in the same way. Consult your prescribing healthcare provider before eliminating any prescription medications. You should feel comfortable with cannabis and how you react to it before reducing other medicines or getting off them. I encourage all of my patients to recognize how cannabis works alongside their medications before considering changes. This knowledge will also help inform your healthcare provider regarding the benefits you experience.

+ **Surprise product recommendation:** High-quality lotions are helpful for insomnia, as they relax muscle tissue in the face and forehead the same way that a massage would. When it is placed on the arms and shoulders, or on the face and thighs, where deep tension is often held over the course of a day, you are likely to feel relaxed enough to fall asleep.

Skipping Doses While Traveling

It is not always possible to travel with THC products. However, it's nothing to worry about: cannabis is building up in your bloodstream over the weeks that you are consuming it, creating a small storage supply, so that products do not necessarily need to be taken every night. In fact, over time, my patients often require less cannabis than they were using before. We know this is true because travelers typically get a couple of nights of good sleep away from home. If you had to skip your cannabis sleep routine for a night or two, you would continue to have sleep benefits. By the third day, your internal supply would be drained.

One fix is to try CBD alternatives for travel days, since it's legal everywhere and can be just as effective. Look for more sedating CBD derivatives, like CBN. It doesn't work quite as well, patients say, as THC-derived products, but it seems to help amplify the body's stores of cannabinoids until you get home.

MEET MARY

My patient Mary has trouble sleeping. She likes the immediacy of CBD tinctures, but she found them to only provide about four to five hours of sleep. She also found that she was developing a tolerance to them and was increasing her dosage frequently.

I explained that there were many other tincture options available that might provide her with better results. We talked about the difference between alcohol tincture versus oil tincture, because I felt she would do better with an oil-based cannabis concentrate. One of my favorites is a CBD product called Rick Simpson Oil: it's like a super-condensed espresso in the coffee world. Mary could switch to that formulation and ensure a longer night's sleep.

Mary has since transitioned to edible candies with sustained benefit for remaining asleep. Occasionally the dispensaries do not carry her preferred choice, and when this happens, she can easily transition to a comparable product.

The Basics of Good Sleep Hygiene

Having a positive experience with cannabis will, in part, depend on how you match your product with your overall sleep hygiene. Cannabis will be more effective when it is paired with optimal sleep hygiene.

+ Set a regular bedtime and rise time: following consistent and more regular sleep schedules avoids periods of sleep deprivation or periods of extended wakefulness during the night.
+ Limit caffeine, especially after lunch.
+ Limit alcohol, especially after dinner. Alcohol is initially sedating, but its high sugar content makes it stimulating as it is metabolized.
+ Your last meal of the day should be at least three hours before bedtime, and skip the late-night snacks. You can eat a healthy and filling meal that's not too large or too small.
+ Nicotine is a stimulant and should be avoided, especially near bedtime.
+ Daytime physical activity promotes a good night's sleep, especially if you can do your exercise four to six hours before bedtime. You may find that exercising too close to bedtime is stimulating.
+ Keep your bedroom cool, dark, comfortable, and quiet. Noise and light can easily disrupt sleep. White noise machines or earplugs can reduce your exposure to noise. Using blackout shades or an eye mask will reduce light. Cover lights on electronic devices that may brighten the room.
+ Avoid television and technology near bedtime. Turn on "nighttime" settings at least an hour before you want to go to sleep to lessen your exposure to bright light before bed.
+ If you wake up in the middle of the night, avoid checking the time. Checking the time increases cognitive arousal and anxiety and prolongs wakefulness.

Monitor Your Sleep Quality

While you should aim for seven to eight hours of sleep every day, including naps, it's not just hitting the right quantity that makes for an official good night's rest.

You also need to take into account your sleep quality, and how satisfied you feel when you wake up. The best way to monitor this is with a sleep journal. You don't have to create a formal document, but ask yourself the following questions when you wake up. If the majority are not pointing to good sleep, discuss your concerns with your healthcare provider, and investigate if cannabis is a good option for you. Your answers may also point you to specific opportunities you can employ to improve your sleep hygiene.

1. Are you at home or elsewhere (vacation, camping, traveling)?
2. Is there anything that you are worrying about (social, family strife, work deadline, etc.)?
3. Are you currently sick (virus, allergies, etc.)?
4. Were you able to have active time outside today (to get fresh air, sun, vitamin D)?
5. In bed, is the temperature comfortable?
6. Is the bedding comfortable and your pillow positioning—the angle of your head and neck—fully relaxing?
7. Did you experience any physical discomfort?
8. Did you snack before, during, or after bedtime? (And what did you eat/drink?)
9. Did you read right before bed?
10. Did you listen to anything at bedtime?
11. Did you shower before going to bed? (This can be a reliable way to help relax tension and clean the body from potentially disruptive and invisible, irritating allergens, like pollen.)
12. Any sexual activity before/during/after bedtime? (All forms of consensual/ pleasurable sexual activity appear to improve sleep quality, duration, and restfulness.)
13. Did you have any arguments before/during/after bedtime? (Unpleasant or uncomfortable thought patterns can set the stage for unpleasant dreams, unsettled sleep, and other sleep interruptions. It is invaluable to create a safe, positive mental retreat prior to sleep.)
14. Are you well hydrated?
15. How did you sleep last night in comparison to a typical night?

16. How many times do you remember waking up?

17. Approximately how long did it take you to fall asleep?

18. Was there any stretch of time (longer than fifteen minutes) when you were awake?

19. For approximately how long were you awake when you wanted to get back to sleep?

20. When you woke up, did you do anything stimulating (look at your phone, listen to music, read, have something to eat)?

21. Did you need to use any product in the night to help you get back to sleep?

22. What time did you use the product?

23. How quickly were you able to get back to sleep after taking the product?

24. Did you experience any sleep interruptions that were unavoidable (kids, partner, alarm, etc.)?

25. How close would you say you got to the sleep you would like?

CHAPTER 8

Headaches

H eadaches are among the most common medical complaints heard from adults. Many people have infrequent headaches and can easily address them with over-the-counter medicines like Tylenol and Advil: the irritation quickly goes away and life goes on. Yet there are just as many who don't find relief from these first-line choices, or they are dealing with a chronic, debilitating, or more painful type of headache. For them, guided cannabis treatments are nothing short of life-changing.

First, let's figure out what type of headache you are dealing with, so we can match the right treatment to your individual needs.

The Most Common Headaches

When a headache occurs as a result of another condition, it is classified as a "secondary headache." These can be caused by a variety of issues, including caffeine withdrawal or dehydration, which are the two most common causes of secondary headaches. Other causes include exhaustion, anxiety, nervousness, illness (long COVID, high blood pressure, dental issues, cysts, tumors, and glaucoma), sinus issues (a cold, allergy, chronic cough), hormonal changes, exercise, posture, physical exertion, medications, and even changes in altitude. Secondary head-aches are typically treated along with the circumstance that brought them on. For instance, when allergy-induced headaches occur, you can treat the headache in a variety of different ways, but if the root cause is still present—like when a dog remains in the room or the pollen outside rages on—the headache is less likely to completely disappear.

Primary headaches occur without a trigger or underlying cause. They tend to be more painful, last longer, and are more disruptive than secondary headaches. These include:

+ **Cluster headaches:** Characterized by the presence of a severe pain on one side of the head, typically around the eyes or temple, accompanied by nasal congestion and a sense of restlessness or agitation. Cluster headaches present with intense pain that develops within a few minutes, and they can last as long as three hours. Traditional treatments include Tylenol, Advil (NSAIDs), amitriptyline, and muscle relaxants.

+ **Tension-type headaches:** Tension headaches are very common and are often linked to emotional stress or physical pain elsewhere on the body. These types of headaches typically present as a dull, pressure headache that waxes and wanes, and the pain occurs on both sides of the head. They are characterized by a gradual onset and mild to moderate intensity with or without facial tenderness. Typically, over-the-counter analgesics like aspirin, Tylenol, or Advil, as well as caffeine, are effective treatments. When tension headaches occur regularly, tricyclic antidepressants like amitriptyline, or muscle relaxants, can be used preventively. Interestingly, antidepressants are often prescribed in an effort to make the suffering less emotionally draining, yet they aren't particularly effective in relieving headaches themselves and often come with adverse effects.

+ **Hemicrania continua:** This type of headache causes continuous pain on one side of your face or head. Women seem to get this more often than men, and they describe it as a dull ache or throb that's interrupted by a more jolting pain. This cycle can occur as much as three to five times a day. Like migraines, they can cause nausea or vomiting, and sensitivity

to noise or light. Symptoms often occur on the painful side of the face and head, including stuffy or runny nose; tearing, redness, or irritation of the eyes; drooping eyelids; and sweating. It is responsive to non-steroidal medicines (NSAIDs) like ibuprofen (Advil), indomethacin (Tivorbex), and diclofenac (Flector, Cambia, Zipsor).

+ **Hypnic headache:** Also known as "alarm clock headache," this type occurs almost exclusively after the age of fifty, and is characterized by episodes of dull head pain, often occurring on both sides of the head, that awaken the sufferer from sleep. Caffeine is considered to be the most effective treatment for hypnic headaches. Even though it sounds counterintuitive, a cup of coffee can help people with hypnic headaches sleep through the night. Preventatively, caffeine and prescribed lithium are the most recommended treatments, followed by indomethacin.

+ **Paroxysmal hemicrania:** Patients with paroxysmal hemicrania typically have one-sided, brief, severe attacks of pain that occur with dizziness, sweating, and heart-rate changes. An individual headache attack usually lasts two to thirty minutes, and can recur as much as eleven to fourteen times a day. Paroxysmal hemicrania most often occurs in women. It can be prevented with regular use of indomethacin, and when symptoms arise, it is treated with the same medication.

+ **Stabbing headache:** Characterized by sudden brief attacks of sharp, jabbing head pain at or around the eyes, or near the temple regions. The stabs last a few seconds and occur at irregular intervals from once to many times each day. Also known as icepick headaches, they can be treated with a range of non-steroidal medicines (NSAIDs).

Focus on Migraines

Migraines are painful and frustrating: they are a recurrent disorder that is difficult to control. Particularly since the beginning of COVID, the prevalence of migraine headaches has only grown. Some people who have had the coronavirus also have a lasting prevalence of migraines, long past the course of the infection. Migraine sufferers often experience headaches on such a regular basis that they can hardly function, professionally or socially. Some patients experience paralyzing pain multiple times a day, every day of the year.

We used to believe that migraines occur when blood vessels are changing diameter, either constricting or relaxing; typically, it's during the relaxing phase when the headache first comes on. Yet we now know that migraines are caused by faulty electrical signals in the brain, causing the activation of pain-sensitive nerves, and leading to inflammation.[1]

Migraines often occur on one side of the head and tend to have a throbbing or pulsating quality. Besides head pain, they are often accompanied by nausea; vomiting; and an extreme sensitivity to light, sound, or smells: any stimulation to sensory nerves causes pain. Some migraines occur with an *aura,* a sensory disturbance like a flash of light or other vision changes. Sufferers may become more sensitive to smells, develop a bad taste in the mouth, or experience numbness and tingling in one hand or on one side of their face. Because of the enhanced sensitivity to stimuli, many people prefer to rest in a dark, quiet room until the migraine passes, although they can last between four and seventy-two hours, and occasionally for days or weeks.

Migraines can come on for no apparent reason, or you may notice that certain factors precede them. These triggers can include stress, menstruation, visual stimuli, scents, weather changes, eating foods high in nitrates (luncheon meats or wine), fasting, sleep disturbances, and sugar substitutes like aspartame.

Typical migraine medicines—analgesics, triptans, anti-inflammatories, anti-emetics, antidepressants, anti-seizure medications, and even Botox—are divided into fast-acting rescue medicines and long-lasting preventatives. The same medications are sometimes used to counteract a migraine or prevent one from happening. However, these medications offer limited localized relief and minimal systemic relaxation, and have side effects including dehydration, fatigue, weakness, and dizziness, all of which can lead to falls and frustration and continued agony. What's more, sufferers have to address migraines urgently, as quickly as they come on, in order to prevent them from becoming severe and further debilitating. Another downside to these medications is that people become very tolerant to them: the most common complaint my migraine patients have is that they have been on five different medicines because, over time, they just don't work anymore.

Although cannabis therapy is rarely discussed during typical primary care visits, my patients have had incredible success with it. In my office, it's not uncommon to hear of migraine sufferers shifting from having migraines multiple times per day to having only one or two per month. Cannabis can treat migraines because it can act as an anti-convulsant, anti-inflammatory, analgesic, and an anti-emetic (prevents vomiting).

Cannabis is an ideal treatment for migraines because of its powerful anti-inflammatory nature. This is also the reason why lotions applied directly to the head or neck where you are experiencing pain are so effective: systemic treatments for inflammation are good, but a strong, local topical can work faster and stronger. In fact, one of the most common applications of topical cannabis is treating migraines. The key is to attack the intracranial tissues. You put the cannabis lotion on your shoulders, neck, or temples, and the cannabinoids will travel to your brain. Only a small amount of cannabinoids are getting into the bloodstream, so even lotions that are THC dominant will not cause a euphoric effect. There are no unpleasant side effects and no dosage ceiling, so users can find the right dosage that brings relief and can stick with it for a long time.

If you're trying to end a migraine quickly, you will want to impact the network of misfiring neurons as directly as possible. Longer-acting, systemic oral options like edibles or tinctures work in a more preventative manner, constantly suppressing painful inflammation so that you can reach a comfortable baseline.

Why Cannabis Works on Headaches

Like some traditional headache medicines, cannabis can be used to help prevent headaches, limit how long they last, and shift the response to managing them when they do arise. Any type of headache can be viewed as having three fundamental components: a cause or source of trouble; a communication channel through which the pain signals may travel; and the destination, where the nerve signals of discomfort are received and interpreted. Cannabis can treat headaches and their associated symptoms at each of these three phases.

At the origination point, or source of pain, cannabis is effective at relaxing muscle tissues, reducing nerve irritation, and lowering inflammation. For instance, cannabis can subdue the muscles inside the lining of arteries, which prevents and treats the contractions that are experienced as migraines. For pain associated with uneven tension of upper body muscles, cannabis soothes muscles to a less tense equilibrium at the muscle of origin.

Cannabis can disrupt the communication of pain signals by connecting with specific receptors found in almost every cell in the body, including nerve cells. In the case of primary headaches, and particularly for migraines, muscular tension, and stress-associated headaches, consumed cannabis molecules interact with these same receptors and exert therapeutic effects by dialing back the signaling of the nerves that sense or transmit pain signals. This can occur because cannabis has the ability to influence electrical ion shifts at the cellular level to create or dampen electrical signals. These electrical signals transmit or reduce the flow of electrical ions (potassium, calcium, and sodium) inside and out of the cell rapidly, influencing pain signals almost immediately. For instance, when you have a headache, the nerve signaling that alerts you to the fact that you have pain occurs in predictable ways. Charged molecules are released and kick-start a chain reaction that sends the headache signal along a set of nerves to the topmost part of the spinal cord. There, a second electrical signal is sent to a different region of the brain, which identifies the headache sensation. Along the way, other regions of the brain receive copycat signals and interpret discomfort, attach related memories, and trigger emotions like frustration, anger, anxiety, and fixation. At each point in the nerve's electrical transmission, cannabis can dampen the strength of the signal. The result is that you experience a softened perception of the intensity of pain, both locally and systemically. Locally, it subdues the signals of discomfort and reduces regional inflammation in the head. Systemically, the presence of cannabis molecules reduces the body's overall stress response; amplifies signals of comfort and satisfaction; and through the diminishing of neural signaling, creates what is often described as a "vacation" or "break" from discomfort. And when headaches happen to come with other unpleasant symptoms, such as nausea, muscular tension, and anger or frustration, cannabis can address those symptoms, too, impacting the electrical nerve signaling in a similar fashion.

The final stop on the headache pathway is the brain. Over time, the repeated transmission of pain signals to the brain is interpreted as durable suffering and can leave a lasting psychological impression. After years of consistent suffering, those with chronic headaches often identify themselves as someone who will never get better, whose life and confidence is limited, and they lose hope. Cannabis's positive effects on the memory center in the brain can diminish the nagging presence of pain by shifting one's focus and recall of distress to comfort.

The Same Relief, but Different

Cannabis works in many of the same targeted ways as traditional pharmaceuticals, and it also works on a much broader scale, touching a variety of receptors at the same time, which is unlike any medicine on the market. For headaches, it is almost like having multiple types of medications working simultaneously. Cannabis acts as a pain reliever, mood stabilizer, anti-inflammatory, and anti-anxiety medication. This can mean that your headaches resolve faster, while you are treating other symptoms.

Traditional NSAID headache medicines act on prostaglandins, which are molecules that control processes including inflammation, blood flow, and nerve transmission. Cannabinoids also act on prostaglandins, while having other powerful effects on even stronger inflammatory agents called *cytokines*. Antidepressants that are used to treat headaches act by increasing serotonin, particularly at 5-HT1 receptors. Cannabinoids act on the same 5-HT1 receptors and also increase serotonin in other ways.[2]

On the largest scale, cannabis is engaging with the full spectrum of the brain's natural neurotransmitter receptors, including dopamine, noradrenaline, glutamate, acetylcholine, GABA, and the opiates. In effect, it has the potential to recalibrate the brain toward optimal health.

Treating Headaches with Cannabis

Once you have identified which type of headache you suffer from, treating it with cannabis is easy. For some headaches, the opportunity to quash the pain early, before it travels to new areas of the head, or before the pain grows, or before it becomes intractable, can make the difference between function and failure. In this case, it is critical to know both your typical pattern of headache and also how the headache responds to different formulations of cannabis. Some headaches are less prone to expansion or variability of intensity, and instead are more persistent and monotonous. In the same way, understanding the match of product and pain is critical to lasting relief.

Cannabis is a very effective antidote for most headaches, but not all. It will not always address the underlying causes of secondary headaches. For instance, with the two most common causes of secondary headaches—dehydration and caffeine withdrawal—cannabis is only marginally effective, and because of its dehydrating properties, might in fact make you feel worse. In this instance, you may be better off with Tylenol or Advil, which are powerful anti-inflammatories that can be used as a first-line headache treatment with secondary headaches. With headaches caused by masses, including tumors inside the skull or around the neck and shoulder region, cannabis may offer an overall sense of comfort, but will not relieve the pressure of the mass in time to thwart the headache. However, as you'll learn in chapter fifteen, I have worked with patients who have successfully used cannabis to shrink and even eliminate tumors.

For chronic and/or primary headaches, cannabis can be used as a first-line treatment. It will easily replace over-the-counter medications like Advil and Tylenol, which have particular concerns and long-term effects, especially for people with organ sensitivities (kidney, stomach, liver). There aren't dramatic long-term consequences that we know of yet with cannabis.

+ **Onset timing:** Typically, my patients want fast relief for their headaches, and cannabis can be just as fast-acting as other traditional medications, depending on the method of consumption. Topicals and inhalants are often recommended because their effect is almost instantaneous. There are some edibles, including quick-acting drinks, and sublinguals that are rapidly effective; gummies or candies would not be a good choice for fast treatment of headaches.

+ **Short-acting versus longer-lasting:** Inhalants and topicals will not provide a sustained effect over time. You may need to reapply lotions regularly or consume inhalants frequently to achieve relief through the day. Or you can take edibles daily, preferably at different times each day, to provide an effective, preventative effect. Staggering your routine in terms of product and timing will help you avoid building tolerance.

+ **Euphoric/non-euphoric:** CBD is currently believed to be a little bit stronger of a systemic anti-inflammatory. THC also has strong anti-inflammatory action, and its euphoric nature also soothes a layer of discomfort that is more emotional or psychological, on top of its effects at reducing regional inflammation. THC provides a layer of distraction so that you can temporarily forget about the pain as well as allows you to focus on more pleasant thoughts.

+ **Compare products:** Compare the products containing specific terpenes and flavonoids to the master list in chapter one to make sure you are getting the benefits you are looking for. I believe that terpenes and flavonoids may offer more nuanced control of headaches, but it has not yet been fully explored in rigorous scientific studies how individuals respond to particular compounds over time.

+ **Product recommendation #1—lotions:** Most headaches, including migraines, seem to be amenable to topical treatments. This is a powerful alternative if you are already treating other chronic illnesses systemically with cannabis, and in circumstances for which traditional anti-inflammatories are discouraged. To be able to apply a cream on the neck, temples, or shoulders and abate a headache feels miraculous. I recommend going with as strong (cannabinoid-dense) a formulation as possible. As time goes on, a less cannabinoid-dense topical may provide enough relief. In general, it is less important to focus on either high THC or CBD products. The most effective lotions will often be a mixture of both, or a product that is either high in THC or CBD that is also rich in terpenes.

+ **Product recommendation #2—humidified cannabinoids:** If you want fast-acting relief without the irritation or heat of vaporized products, humidified cannabis is an effective alternative. Instead of breathing in smoke or vapor, you can breathe humidified cannabis via a nebulizer. This is particularly helpful for sinus headaches and headaches related to infections, as cannabinoids have evidence to show that they have antiviral, antimicrobial, and antibacterial properties.[3]

+ **Cannabis and medications:** Adding cannabis products will make your existing prescription regimen work better for headaches caused by migraines, muscle pains, and anxiety. Marrying two types of treatment is often more effective than each individually. Cannabis is also often found to eliminate the side effects of headache medications. Do not stop taking prescription medications without fully consulting your prescribing healthcare provider. You should feel comfortable with cannabis and how it might make you feel before you entertain reducing other medicines or getting off them.

MEET HAROLD

Harold came to see me when he was seventy-three years old. He had already been diagnosed with heart disease and frequent migraines. Harold told me that as he has gotten older, the preventive migraine treatments he has tried, including propranolol, amitriptyline, and over-the-counter medicines, are no longer effective. He has become less comfortable with migraine medicines such as sumatriptan, which make him feel unsteady.

I suggested that he try something completely different to prevent migraines: cannabis lotion. I explained that, initially, he could use the lotion every day to build up effective levels in his bloodstream. This strategy would be both therapeutic to rescue him from his headaches and help prevent future discomfort. After two or three weeks, he could switch to applying the lotion more intermittently without losing the benefit of prevention.

A few weeks later, Harold gave me a call. Not only had he been able to eliminate the pills from his daily routine, the severity and frequency of his migraines dropped considerably. As soon as Harold feels a headache beginning, he knows to apply the lotion to his temples. He then reapplies lotion periodically through the day, and maintains relief with no further need for either preventative or rescue prescription medications.

CHAPTER 9

Neurodegenerative Diseases: Dementia, Alzheimer's, and Parkinson's

W hen the brain is healthy, we can move easily, recall memories, and maintain good attention. The gradual loss of these functions is often interpreted as a normal part of aging. Yet we in the medical community know that this is not always the case: you can maintain a healthy brain for your entire life. We also know that, under challenging conditions, the brain is suspect to illness and degradation, just like any other organ in the body.

The present understanding of neurodegenerative diseases, including Alzheimer's disease, dementia, and Parkinson's disease, is that they often occur alongside brain cell death, which can be caused by many factors. The first is a mucking up, or a clogging, that results from either malnourishment or an accumulation of debris, which coincides with the destruction or degradation of nerve cells in the brain. When nerves are supported by good blood flow that delivers quality nutrition, and a healthy cellular structure, they will thrive, strengthen, grow, and multiply. Yet nerves can become malnourished due to poor blood flow. Poor nutrition directly affects the *neural sheath*, the fatty layer that surrounds the nerves in the brain, which is meant to keep signals transmitting without mis-firing. However, malnourished, frayed nerves are prone to misfiring, causing cognitive and physical challenges.

Cannabis is thought to assist the flow of nutrition to the brain by improv-ing arterial blood flow by lowering inflammation and relaxing the smooth muscle tissue that lines all arteries. This is done by enhancing the release of a naturally occurring chemical, nitric oxide, along arterial walls.[1] It can also enhance brain growth factors. Low doses of cannabis molecules initially suppress brain-derived neurotropic factors (BDNF), which are needed to provide nutrition to brain cells.[2] When BDNF is suppressed, the brain has a built-in feedback mechanism to increase production. However, when there is an excessive amount of cannabis available, it can handicap brain growth, as this feedback mechanism cannot keep up with the demand.

Cannabis is thought to support the well-being of both the neural sheath and the nerves themselves. For every sequence of nerves, the stimulation of cannabi-noid receptors where two nerves come together activates the originating nerve.[3] This activation enhances normal cell functions and encourages the nerve to thrive. When your brain is full of healthy nerve connections, it is able to correctly process sensory input, higher cognitive function, and often, deeper analytical skills. It can also foster a healthier response to the buildup of plaque or tangles of proteins in the brain that may be impeding the brain's ability to function optimally. Ultimately through these mechanisms, cannabis can help orchestrate the reversal of some structural damage and provide an environment that is better able to nourish the cells so that they continue working.

Nerve cells can also wither away when there is a lack of activation from their supportive networks. One interesting theory is that the mucking up of brain tis-sues may be due to a failure in the cleanup processes, resulting in a buildup of certain proteins and plaque. Fragile nerve cells depend on their neighboring cells' electrical activating signals to remain alive and thriving. These neighbors include *microglial cells*, whose job is to dispose of the brain's waste through the lymphatic system during sleep.[4] Enhancing the activation of microglial cells promotes the removal of this accumulation, and has been shown to occur at specific frequencies of light and sound,[5] as well as in the presence of cannabinoids.

Some brain illnesses stem from poor diet, poor exercise, poor physical health, stress, anxiety, depression, mental illness, and especially poor sleep. Cannabinoids can assist us with addressing many of these issues. They can help us get better sleep, which reduces stress and provides the opportunity for the brain to adequately process the day's activities, thoughts, feelings, and memories. This full reset every night is not only important for maintaining good physical and mental health, but for making healthy choices when it comes to diet and exercise. And by maintaining a more stable mood, you can enrich social relationships, which we know is essential for maintaining healthy brain function.[6]

The body's immune cells, toxic chemicals, and some pharmaceuticals can also contribute to poor brain function. Endocannabinoid molecules easily react to harmful toxins that we don't want in our system. In fact, they work just the same way as the antioxidants we gain from eating colorful fruits and vegetables. When we take in additional external cannabinoids and their related flavonoids, we are increasing our supply of antioxidants.[7] Cannabis is thought to absorb some forms of toxicity: the shape of cannabinoid molecules acts like tiny floating shields that protect us from the ravaging effects of daily ultraviolet radiation.[8] A different mechanism also protects us from naturally occurring internal toxins such as oxidative stress and an overactive immune system.[9]

Lastly, some brain illnesses have a genetic component. When this occurs, brain cell death is often linked to damage of the *basal ganglia*, a series of connected structures in the brain related to movement and learning.[10] This area is densely packed with cannabinoid receptors, whether they are appropriately functioning or not, determined by your genetic makeup. While more studies need to be done, some researchers believe that cannabis therapies may have a direct impact on preserving function in this area by helping the brain release the chemical dopamine,[11] or addressing damage. What's more, cannabis directly affects your epigenetic expression, where the thriving activity of healthy cells reduces your risk of developing genetic issues in this area of the brain.[12]

For these reasons, cannabis may be a therapy that addresses the root causes of poor brain health, particularly in the three most common areas that afflict adults: dementia/Alzheimer's disease, vascular disease, and Parkinson's disease. In fact, it's not merely the least bad option. It's a great option.

The conditions reviewed in this chapter are devastating, not only for the person who receives the diagnosis, but for the whole family. The trajectory for each of these illnesses is ultimately catastrophic. What's more, traditional treatments are sometimes worse than the disease. Many of the traditional medications change the sufferer's personality, as well as their ability to express their needs and interact with others. The existing approach to care falls far short of the way most people wish to spend their remaining years, and it can have lasting ripple effects for the rest of the family.

In contrast, guided cannabis therapies can offer an entirely different trajectory, from the initial diagnosis to end of life. It can provide the ability to remain calm during the earliest stages following a diagnosis, so that people can make good choices going forward. Over the course of the illness, cannabis provides a welcome stability and a consistent source of comfort without a hurricane of side effects and personality distortions. And as you've just learned, it may be able to reverse some of the damage caused, extending brain function.

My typical patient with brain health issues is generally frustrated that the medical system has not met their expectations and is tired of orienting their remaining years around debilitating medication side effects. Instead, they are looking for a therapy that can provide consistent outcomes that can bring back a sense of normalcy to their daily life. For these diseases, the promise of guided cannabis therapies has met, and often exceeded, their expectations.

You Can Forget About the Fear of "Killing Brain Cells"

Despite its reputation for "killing brain cells," cannabis is not the culprit it has been made out to be. Concerns about cannabis's harmful properties—causing schizophrenia, destroying brain cells, making the user dim-minded and lazy, and a stepping-stone to other, more dangerous drugs—first gained traction in the 1930s and has been periodically reinforced for sociopolitical agendas. In fact, this reputation is in stark contrast to the scientific research, which has always been, and continues to be, largely neutral or supportive of its efficacy.

Science has shown that cannabis use is not going to cause any of the above conditions, nor is it going to lead to dementia, long-term forgetfulness, or memory issues. In fact, in terms of brain health, the benefits of using cannabis include reversing the cognitive deterioration that can occur as related to the risks of everyday life. By promoting better sleep, enhancing calmness, and lowering inflammation with cannabis, you are naturally enhancing *neurogenesis*, the creation of new brain cells, which leads to having a more robust brain and developing stronger neural networks.[13] Cannabis also provides the necessary nutrients and activation of the brain's support systems to further enhance neurogenesis.[14] We also know that the daily life of someone suffering from neurodegenerative diseases is full of anxiety, depression, and sleeplessness, all of which are linked to worsening dementia. CBD research has shown that it can help increase neurogenesis in mice dealing with unpredictable stress.[15]

Neurogenesis is believed to be a foundational concept for reversing cell damage and even curing the diseases covered in this chapter. Cannabis may indeed be part of the solution, through its ability to systematically and continuously stop brain cell death and increase the amount of new brain cells. At this time more studies are needed. However, I do feel confident in suggesting cannabis therapies if you have received a confirmed diagnosis. Literally, your brain health has everything to gain.

However, too much of anything rarely leads to positive outcomes. We do know that in the short term, excessive THC-based cannabis levels in the body prevent normal nerve function. In the long term, it can also affect normal nerve development, leading to a slowing of nerve-to-nerve signaling and a reduction in the overall thriving of nerves. The resulting interruption in speedy processing can look similar to neurodegenerative decline.

If you are trying THC products to address your brain health and not seeing results, it is possible that you are taking too much. Try lower levels of product or switching to CBD-dominant choices.

Dementia and Alzheimer's Disease

Dementia is a broad term that is used to characterize a decline in cognition involving at least one of the following areas of brain function that can interfere with the activities of daily life and overall independence:[16]

+ Complex attention
+ Executive function
+ Language
+ Learning and memory
+ Perceptual-motor skills
+ Social cognition

There are many forms of dementia, including Alzheimer's disease. Some dementias result from illness or injury; others appear with normal aging. Typical symptoms beyond the impairments listed above include agitation, delusions, and acting-out behaviors.

There is no existing cure for Alzheimer's or other dementias. However, cannabinoids may make a difference. As cannabinoids are strong antioxidants, they protect the brain from damage, including oxidative stress. They are also shown to be an effective strategy in animal studies for creating new brain cells via neurogenesis, as well as stronger nerve-to-nerve connections, which help brain cells thrive.[17] Lastly, the improved functioning of these cells means that they are prone to remain free of the accumulated plaques and debris associated with Alzheimer's and dementia. Studies show that with cannabis on board, the brain plaques in patients with dementia/Alzheimer's disease seem to be deteriorating as the microglial cells are activating, and blood flow is improving.[18]

There is also clinical data that highlights the success of using cannabis to address the symptoms of dementia, making these debilitating illnesses easier to live with. One study showed a significant drop in behavioral disturbances in people with Alzheimer's disease when they were taking the THC prescription medication dronabinol.[19] This is an important finding, as we know that people suffering from dementias are likely to be depressed and aggressive. But with cannabis on board, these same people are less unhappy and can feel more relaxed. They're sleeping better. They're less agitated. By lowering panic and increasing attention, day-to-day life activities can become pleasurable, where calmness begets more calmness instead of anxiety begetting more anxiety.

Treating dementia and Alzheimer's disease with cannabis has been shown to be an effective strategy with fewer debilitating side effects than the traditional medicines. The one medication on the market that treats Alzheimer's disease is aducanumab, which may help reduce the plaques associated with this disease. Because this medication is new to the marketplace, we don't yet know how cannabis use will impact its efficacy. Another type of medication commonly prescribed are the cholinesterase inhibitors donepezil, galantamine, and rivastigmine. These medications address the behavioral issues that surround dementia and seek to improve cognition, rather than targeting the cause of the disease. These medicines are generally found to be unpalatable because of their strong sedating side effects, as well as increased risk of stroke and death.[20] Cannabis is thought to inhibit the enzymes that break down the brain chemical acetylcholine, making it more available, which is the same action as these medications without the risky side effects. Taken together, they may augment each other.

Mixing Technology with Cannabis for Better Brain Health

Scientific interpretations are often made through indirect association: if A causes B, and B causes C, it's logical to think that A causes C. In studies from the McGovern Institute for Brain Research at MIT, when the microglial cells in animal brains were exposed to flashes of lights and sounds and at a steady rate of speed, their existing Alzheimer's plaques were reduced by more than half.[21] If cannabis can also stimulate microglial cells, it seems logical that it can affect brain plaques in a similar fashion.

There are apps right on your phone that can provide the same light and sound stimulation at specific frequencies known to reduce Alzheimer's plaques. Search for "binaural" in the App Store or Google Play to test these for yourself. My patients have found improved sleep and increased focus, attention, and restfulness by combining them with their cannabis use.

Treating the Stages of Alzheimer's Disease/Dementias

Alzheimer's disease and other forms of dementia typically occur over a long period of time. In fact, one can be in the earliest stages of these diseases for up to twenty years. Cannabis can be an effective strategy through every stage in different ways, and one can continue treatment to the end of one's life, albeit in different forms. While we don't know if it can fully make Alzheimer's disease and dementia go away, it can make your life more comfortable. It offers a smoothing of an otherwise difficult daily experience with life over a long period of time. It makes the emotional struggles more tolerable, and most importantly, dials back the frustration and anxiety of forgetfulness.

I see patients at every stage of the disease, including those without a formal diagnosis. A typical patient may be in their early sixties with a family history of dementia. For instance, Sue came to my office with a real sense of both fear and hopelessness. She was convinced that she was losing her cognitive function, even though she had not received a formal diagnosis. However, Sue told me that she's been increasingly forgetful. She periodically finds herself on the phone forgetting what she's talking about, or reading a paragraph in a book and has no idea what she just read. I recommended that Sue get a full cognitive workup from a neurologist, who could confirm or allay her fears. Until she had a formal diagnosis, I suggested a variety of choices that would feel both empowering and treat her forgetfulness. I explained that making cannabis a regular part of her daily life would help her sleep more comfortably, and feel less anxious during the daytime; this is important because people often mistake the forgetfulness of dementia with the overwhelming thoughts that stem from anxiety, distraction, fatigue, and poor sleep. At the same time, the inflammatory effects that make someone prone to dementia would be actively reduced via cannabis consumption. To start, I recommended that Sue take a low-dose combination THC/CBD edible at night, an hour before she goes to sleep, to relieve her anxiety and ensure a good night's rest. This nighttime regimen will, over time, create the buildup effect so that it would carry her through her daytime routine, with a steady relief of her anxiety. I assured her that, sometimes, addressing those two factors is all it takes to restore cognitive function.

Once there is a formal diagnosis, you can attempt to slow the progression of the disease by tapping into the endocannabinoid system, which helps clean the muck building up in your brain. Cannabis is stimulating new cell growth, while healing damaged tissues and preventing outside damage by lowering inflammation.

On the other end of the spectrum, I often speak with a caregiver for a spouse or parent who has dementia, who is at their wit's end because their parent is very angry and aggressive. In this situation, I first explain that behavioral issues like these occur in part because nonverbal patients are often confused and disoriented. They're constantly badgered by people who they no longer recognize. They're rarely comfortable, and they're certainly not sleeping well. I once spoke to Juan, who was so frustrated because his father wouldn't let him touch or bathe him. Without the basics of daily care, Juan's father was becoming increasingly disheveled, to the point where Juan was worried that he would get an infection. Bed sores were appearing, and his father had hand wounds from hitting things. I explained that Juan could offer his father cannabis to help him relax without completely sedating him the way prescription anxiolytics would. I mentioned that adults with dementia often seem childlike, especially with the foods they enjoy. Many of my later-stage patients like Juan's father respond well to THC chocolates: they look forward to their daily candy, and in a very short time start feeling calmer, able to relax, and able to sleep. Over time, they can tolerate assistance with their personal care routines, which will keep them healthier longer. And, when other illnesses inevitably arise, cannabis can mitigate the additional angst so that Juan's father will more easily accept the best appropriate care.

Parkinson's Disease

Our nerves communicate to and from the brain using thousands of synergistic and opposing connections. To flex an arm, for instance, requires multiple nerves to signal various muscle fiber subgroups within the biceps to contract. At the same time, fibers in the triceps must be signaled to relax. If this simultaneous signaling is somewhat off, you might straighten your arm rather than bend it. Most muscles in the body operate similarly in opposing pairs, or in sequential rhythmic pulsing, such as the contractions of the tongue or the digestive system. It is now known that skeletal muscle tissues contain receptors for cannabinoids. At the same time, it's also known that cannabinoid receptor activation affects calcium release within the muscle cells, thereby affecting the muscle's ability to contract. This change in contractility will send signals to the brain that the muscle is contracting with less strength, or give an impression that it is fatigued, perhaps ultimately leading to sleepiness. This is the main reason why people commonly report feeling sleepy when they are taking cannabis products, even when they aren't meant to cause sedation.

Even though the symptoms of Parkinson's disease occur in the body, the misfiring of nerves causes a communication issue in the brain. Parkinson's disease is caused by a deficit of the brain chemical dopamine, typically produced in the *substantia nigra*, found within the basal ganglia. Without the appropriate amount of dopamine, the nerve signaling from the brain to the body is insufficient for smooth muscle function, resulting in movement symptoms including stiffness, poor balance, slowness in movement, and tremors in the hands and/or feet, even at rest. Just as a car may have spits, sputters, or jolts if fuel lines are improperly flowing or functioning, the misfunctioning transmission of dopamine in Parkinson's disease causes some similarly erratic motor manifestations.

There are also non-motor symptoms of the disease, which can include:

+ A drop in blood pressure when standing (orthostatic hypotension)
+ Anxiety
+ Bodily pain
+ Cognitive changes
+ Dementia
+ Dental issues
+ Depression
+ Drooling
+ Gastrointestinal issues
+ Hallucinations or delusions
+ Impulsive behaviors
+ Reduced sense of smell (hyposmia)
+ Sexual dysfunction
+ Skin problems: dry or oily skin, or excessive sweating
+ Sleep disruptions
+ Urinary frequency
+ Vision problems
+ Weight changes

We have seen in scientific study that cannabinoids can improve both the motor and non-motor symptoms of Parkinson's disease. This occurs for a few different reasons. For motor symptoms, cannabis products can help joints act more smoothly by making dopamine more available.[22] As cannabis increases your ability to access sensory input, it refreshes well-worn pathways of the brain in ways that rejuvenate connections and chemistry, for more effective brain signaling. The antioxidant effects of cannabis also help invigorate dopamine levels.[23] Lastly, within a supportive set and setting, cannabis products have been shown to modulate dopamine-related transmission, in ways that promote dopamine release, and potentially ways that limit its release, depending upon whether one takes CBD- or THC-based products. The data is still preliminary but seems to suggest that CBD is more likely to support increased fluidity of movements in Parkinson's patients.[24]

Cannabinoids can treat motor symptoms as well as the non-motor symptoms at the same time. The action of cannabinoids on motor nerves is direct. There are dense cannabinoid receptors on the same areas of the brain that produce dopamine. For non-motor symptoms, the action of cannabinoids is more indirect but no less powerful, enabling deeper sleep, improving moods, allowing for stronger relaxation, and managing pain. It also allows for a refreshed outlook on daily life, escaping the monotony and melancholy of dealing with this physically and emotionally devastating chronic illness.

There is currently no known cure for Parkinson's disease, yet there are a wide variety of treatments that can help manage its symptoms. Your healthcare provider can recommend a particular treatment based on your symptoms, the stage of your disease, your level of functional ability, and the level of physical activity and productivity you are trying to achieve. Traditional Parkinson's medications fall into four main classes. Monoamine oxidase type B (MAO B) inhibitors and amantadine are typically prescribed for those with mild symptoms. Dopamine agonists can improve motor symptoms but carry the highest risk for developing hallucinations. Levodopa is considered to be the most effective, yet it requires the most frequent dosing. Anti-cholinergic drugs are often prescribed to alleviate tremors. The most aggressive side effects of any of these medications are nausea, memory impairment, confusion, and hallucinations.

Cannabis can be used in conjunction with any of these medications. Over time, you may not need as much of the traditional medicine; let your healthcare provider know that you are trying cannabis therapies. In many cases, cannabis is not only compatible with the typical medicines, cannabis makes current Parkinson's medications work better. I use it in concert with Parkinson's medications simply because we are not at a level of confidence with cannabis that we can do without the extra added dopamine. In an ideal world, it seems very clear to me that there's a path where people may be able to consume certain components of cannabis and not depend on other medicines, but we're not there yet.

MEET JOE

My patient Joe used to be a professional dancer. In his late seventies, he was diagnosed with Parkinson's disease. With my help and guided cannabis treatment, Joe is able to dance again. He's not doing the tango or lunging across the dance floor anymore, but he is able to move more fluidly, which is a huge improvement on his quality of life.

Joe was nervous about trying cannabis. He thought of cannabis as a "drug for druggies," but he was willing to give it a try once I explained that while the exact mechanisms as to why cannabis helps those with Parkinson's is still not entirely clear, when we looked at each one of Joe's symptoms, I could see a direct pathway for cannabinoids to help. Cannabis would improve his Parkinson's symptoms, affect the underlying cause, and allow him to be less anxious so that he would be willing to try to move again.

After the first few weeks, he reported that he was feeling a little bit more connected with mobility in a way that never happened with any other medicine. Joe started walking around the block. He was able to do a little bit of a jig on his daughter's wedding day. That small taste of a life that is not frozen was more than he ever hoped for, as he had not found it with other medicines or treatments.

Cannabis Treatment Regimens for Neurodegenerative Diseases

When it comes to neurodegenerative disease, the decision for which type of products to use will vary depending on one's physical limitations and the stage of the disease. For example, with Parkinson's disease, there is an increasing loss of facility of movement. Some people with Alzheimer's disease or Parkinson's can't feed themselves or open a medicine bottle. For these people, pills and edibles could be effective choices if a caregiver is available. Many end-stage patients enjoy smoking, because they can get a strong dose of effective medicine in a short amount of time with minimal effort. The typical long-term downsides of smoking are unlikely to manifest in the years following a neurodegenerative diagnosis.

+ **Onset timing:** Moderate doses of rapidly acting formulations, preferably a CBD-dominant mixture with THC. The dosage will likely increase over time when it's no longer as effective on a daily basis.

+ **Short-acting versus longer-lasting:** In general, most patients with brain health issues find long-lasting "baseline" medication choices effective to avoid mood fluctuations. However, there will be times when you may want, or require, instant gratification. While neurodegenerative diseases are ever present, your short-term, day-to-day experience can be improved.

+ **Daytime or nighttime:** For less severe symptoms that are overall less debilitating, persistent, or at least tolerable, nighttime dosage is most common. For severe symptoms—when you are no longer able to perform the activities of daily living (bathing, dressing, feeding, transitioning from sitting to standing, toileting)—daytime dosing may be necessary.

+ **Euphoric/non-euphoric:** For those with predominant symptoms of mental discomfort, euphoric choices that are higher in THC are typically preferred. For physical concerns, CBD has been shown to be more effective.

+ **Compare products:** Compare the products containing specific terpenes and flavonoids to the master list in chapter one to make sure you are getting the benefits you are looking for. Alongside the major cannabinoids, terpenes and flavonoids may offer more nuanced control of certain side effects related to brain health, but it has not yet been fully explored in rigorous scientific studies.

+ **Product recommendation #1—edibles and tinctures:** In order to treat neurodegenerative conditions, cannabinoids need to penetrate the basal ganglia consistently. I have found that the most efficient and effective systemic options for these conditions are tinctures and edibles, particularly the candy options because they can be used consistently over prolonged periods of time. Interestingly, one of the memories that stays with us through cognitive decline is the brain's reward signaling that happens when we eat sweets. The unconscious pleasure of sweets, the insatiable appetite for them, and the memory of their appeal are actually three phenomena governed in part by the endocannabinoid system. In addition to the benefits they offer, the process of taking the medicine itself becomes quite pleasurable.

+ **Product recommendation #2—nebulzation:** Breathing in cannabis steam is also an opportunity for those who have dementia to safely benefit from lung distribution. Humidified air is well tolerated, generally easy to administer by face mask, and rapidly acting. The advantages of nebulizers over vaporizers, which also have rapid onset and system penetration, include the cool temperatures and diluted potency, which are often a better match for older adults who are frequently more sensitive to extreme sensations.

CHAPTER 10

Seizures

A seizure occurs when there is a misfiring of neurons, or excessive or asynchronous nerve discharges in such a way that normal nerve firing (and, therefore, normal physical behavior) is disrupted. When this occurs, it can cause a loss of focus, muscle control, and consciousness that can last for just seconds to a few minutes, even for days on end.

Seizures can be painful, violent, and alarming, as well as confusing and somewhat embarrassing. Some of the more benign seizures can manifest simply as staring spells or occasional sensory hallucinations, such as noticing a random or peculiar smell or taste. It's not uncommon, even with less intense seizures, to have muscle cramping or progressive loss of muscle tone that can occur in any muscle group—from the muscles surrounding the eyes to the complete back. Occasionally, people soil themselves.

Many people experience more than one type of seizure, which are defined by their intensity and frequency. *Focal seizures* initially involve only a portion of the brain and may spread to neighboring or remote regions. This variety can cause minimal symptoms: a small twitch or a bad taste in your mouth. *Generalized seizures* affect a broader region of the body compared to focal seizures. The experience can range from losing focus for a few seconds to experiencing strong muscle contractions (either going limp or stiffening) and involuntary shaking and screaming. The worst instances, known as *grand mal seizures*, can result in death: sufferers can inadvertently choke on their tongue; drown in their own saliva; or jerk with such vigor that they knock themselves out, cause bodily harm, or incur traumatic brain damage.

When seizures occur, the recovery following an incident can be almost as bad as the initial experience. The recovery process is physically and emotionally exhausting, and it frequently leaves the sufferer in an incapacitated state. It can take up to a couple of days to get back to normal functioning following even the mildest seizures, affecting work, social relationships, and many other aspects of daily life.

Some people have experienced seizures since birth. Others develop seizures later in life, prompted by outside forces like a head injury; an illness causing a high fever; stroke; a reaction to medication; a response to a trigger like stress, alcohol, or lack of sleep; a temporary deprivation of oxygen that interrupts the normal functioning and signaling of cells; or the presence of a foreign body in the brain, such as a tumor. When seizures become a recurrent problem, this is known as *epilepsy*. Epilepsy is considered to be a disease associated with lasting derangement of normal brain function. While it is similar to neurodegenerative diseases in that the insult occurs in the brain, and it may arise from a variety of genetic, structural, metabolic, immune, infectious, or unknown causes, the mechanism is completely different. Instead of faulty nerves that are degrading, seizures occur when healthy nerves misfire their electrical signals.

There are unprovoked asymptomatic seizures that can occur spontaneously, or following a systemic illness or exposure (like toxic chemicals), or a brain injury. There are also symptomatic seizures, where you may be able to recognize when one is coming on. Some of the symptoms that can precede a seizure include:

+ Anxiousness
+ Auditory hallucinations
+ Biting your tongue
+ Confusion
+ Dizziness
+ Headache
+ Loss of bladder or bowel control
+ Mood changes

+ Nausea
+ Rapid blinking or eye movements
+ Teeth clenching
+ Vision changes
+ Weakness

Treating Seizures with Cannabis

The management of seizures is typically focused on five main objectives: prevention, minimizing seizure intensity and severity, minimizing the side effects from medication, reducing the intensity and duration of post-seizure recovery, and improving overall quality of life. The mainstay of therapy for seizures involves administration of one or more anti-epileptic medications, and unfortunately, approximately one-third of patients with epilepsy have seizures that are resistant to anti-epileptic medications.[1] Understandably, many dissatisfied sufferers look to alternative medical practices, including acupuncture, meditation, chiropractic, or psychedelics for potential treatment, with few positive results.[2] Diet, exercise, and nutrition have not been shown to help much either.

However, cannabis may be a viable alternative, and for many, the singular effective treatment. A detailed description of cannabis uses for treating seizures was published in 1843 by W. B. O'Shaughnessy.[3] More recently, studies have shown that cannabinoids decrease the release of excitatory brain chemicals in the central nervous system, which is how they prevent seizures from occurring and lower the intensity of seizures when they occur.[4]

Seizures are one of the few diagnoses where the traditional medical community accepts cannabis as an effective therapeutic agent and has seen dramatic improvement and patient satisfaction with its use. The reason for this acceptance is purely data driven. There have been many studies that have shown that cannabis can treat seizures: on the cellular level in petri dishes, in animal models, and in anecdotal human data. For example, in 1949, one study showed that THC worked as a treatment for epilepsy on five children, where one became seizure free, one was almost seizure free, and three had no change.[5] In 1975, another case was recorded in the medical journals in which a man with epilepsy, who had failed on traditional therapies, added cannabis, and the combination made him seizure-free.[6] Since those early days, there have been many human trials that have confirmed cannabis's efficacy, in both THC and CBD formulations. For instance, in 2004, there was a study of 136 patients that showed dramatic, positive results using cannabinoid products alone, without other anti-epileptic drugs.[7] Other published case reports have confirmed reduced seizure intensity as well as fewer provoked seizures when cannabis is added to traditional seizure medications.

Over the years, I have treated hundreds of epileptic patients and have seen dramatic, positive results. Many of my patients report up to 80 percent less seizure activity. Most have previously tried all kinds of seizure medicine combinations, yet they still complain that these medicines seldom provide the relief they are looking for. Either the medications don't work, or the side effects from them are not manageable. Oftentimes, traditional seizure medicines may be overly sedating or have unbearable side effects such as diarrhea, dizziness, or fatigue. Worse, some of these medications have been found to cause fertility issues in men and women, and for pregnant women, they may affect the fetus. They can also cause low vitamin absorption, directly affect mood leading to worsening symptoms of depression and anxiety, and even potentially increase the risk for self-harm.

While the connection between cannabis use and lower seizure rates seems to be favorable, it is not absolutely so. In some cases, connections have been made between cannabis use and increased seizure activity. One explanation for these potentially confusing findings is that those who use cannabis to help manage their seizures may have an occasional breakthrough seizure resulting from a trigger or other illness. Or it may be that as the systemic cannabinoid levels fall between doses, in someone with epilepsy, the lower level of cannabinoids is insufficient.

Outside of cannabis, the most successful seizure medications for both prevention and treatment are classified as anti-epileptics, including levetiracetam (Keppra), carbamazepine (Carbatrol, Tegretol), phenytoin (Dilantin, Phenytek), oxcarbazepine (Trileptal), lamotrigine (Lamictal), phenobarbital, and lorazepam (Ativan). They all work somewhat differently, yet all bind either with the brain's GABA receptors, the voltage-dependent ion channels in the body, or by affecting the amounts of other brain chemicals like glutamate or the amino acid aspartate. GABA stands for *gamma-aminobutyric acid*, which is a brain chemical that manages the brain's electrical connections, and when it is at the right levels ensures a steady and smooth flow. In essence, it is our body's natural medicine for stopping seizure activity. It is thought that enhancing GABA levels may boost mood, relax the nervous system, reduce pain, and perhaps affect seizure activity.

The anti-seizure effect of cannabis is powerful, often yielding success when other treatments fail, and boosting results of traditional therapies dramatically. Cannabinoid molecules are thought to attach to the same GABA receptors, dampening faulty nerve signals and repairing them. Cannabinoids don't necessarily shut down systems with as much intensity or "force" as pharmaceuticals do. Instead, they act as an effective anti-convulsant that can both decrease acute instances and prevent them.

Historically, matching the right medications to seizure type was important. However, no matter the cause, guided cannabis works. Cannabis is user-controlled, with appealing forms of administration, convenient options for scheduling, and almost all pleasurable without adverse effects. It can be used preventively to reduce seizure frequency, and as needed to reduce intensity. There are also people who take cannabis at night because they want better sleep, if in fact poor sleep is one of their triggers.

Choosing Between Prescription Cannabis and Dispensary Cannabis

With FDA approved use, seizure sufferers have lots of treatment options. Your doctor may prescribe Epidiolex, which is a pharmaceutical CBD formulation that delivers medication in traditional pill forms. Sometimes this is the most cost-effective option, and it will be covered by a health insurance plan. What's more, you are guaranteed to have a safe, reliable source of cannabinoids.

Yet the vast majority of my patients with seizures eventually want to treat themselves with cannabis that is not in pill form or not produced by a pharmaceutical company. The dose of CBD that is delivered in Epidiolex is pretty high, and there are plenty of people who have seizures that would require a far lower dosage. What's more, Epidiolex does not have THC in its product, and the presence of THC and/or other cannabinoids along with CBD makes the CBD more effective at reducing seizures. Lastly, some people simply prefer consuming cannabis products from dispensaries over traditional medicine. They like the idea that they are taking a medicine in candy form or as raw plant materials. They like the control of using products based on their schedule rather than their doctor's.

In the end, the decision between these two very good options is entirely up to you.

Cannabis Regimens for Seizures

In addition to matching seizure timing with onset and duration of cannabis products, the dosage of cannabis seems to correlate with the severity of seizure presentation. The more powerful the seizures, the more effective larger doses of cannabinoids will be.

+ **Onset timing:** The prescription for controlling seizures will vary depending on the baseline seizure frequency and the severity. Some of my patients have sporadic seizures that are predictable and come with warnings, and others have consistent experiences, yet they cannot tell in advance when a seizure is coming. For the former, fast-acting cannabis choices are effective to control the seizures without posing meaningful interference with daily routines. For the latter, longer-lasting products are more likely to cushion a day's risk of recurrences.

+ **Short-acting versus longer-lasting:** For cases of consistent seizure activity, regimens that incorporate longer-lasting results, such as edibles and suppositories, may provide more relief. Many of my patients have adopted a daily ritual of taking an edible each night, microdosing with low-dose mints every few hours at work, or applying a patch each morning.

+ **Daytime or nighttime:** Some individuals prefer the privacy and seclusion of medicating only at night. For preventing seizures, my patients seem to prefer nighttime administration. Others have found that CBD-dominant products work effectively without the potential distraction of euphoric effects, and they often choose to medicate during the daytime.

+ **Euphoric/non-euphoric:** If you are dealing with seizures and depression, euphoric choices offer an opportunity to address both issues at once. The pharmaceutical option Epidiolex is a purified form of CBD, which avoids the euphoric effects.

+ **Compare products:** Compare the products containing specific terpenes and flavonoids to the master list in chapter one to make sure you are getting the benefits you are looking for. We believe that terpenes and flavonoids may offer more nuanced control of seizures, but it has not yet been fully explored in rigorous scientific studies.

+ **Product recommendation:** Fast-acting suppositories. During the digestion and absorption processes, we lose a portion of cannabinoids, and it takes longer for the body to reap the benefits of the treatment. For seizures, both the timing and precision of dosing is critical. When you can administer it through the rectum, you're delivering cannabis directly into the bloodstream. Suppositories offer a way to get a high volume of cannabis into your system in a way that's not terribly unpleasant. Traditional seizure medications also come as rectal suppositories, so this delivery system will not be unfamiliar. Don't worry that the dosage will cause an overwhelming euphoria. Instead, many people experience a pleasant feeling of warmth that pervades the body (like sitting next to a warm fire on a cold day), without an abundance of euphoria, even if the suppositories contain high levels of THC.

+ **Cannabis and medications:** Adding cannabis products to your existing prescription regimen can make your seizure medication work better. Do not stop taking prescription medications without fully consulting your prescribing healthcare provider. You should feel comfortable with cannabis and how it might make you feel before you entertain reducing other medicines or getting off them.

MEET TONY

Tony is one of my most memorable patients. He suffered a traumatic brain injury while working in a construction site. Ever since, and without a clear sense of his triggers, Tony's body would freeze up in stiffness, his gaze would soften, and he would be unable to work for at least a day or two following the episode. Before Tony came to see me, he had tried six different traditional seizure medications with limited success. Often, they would work for only a few months, and they had terrible side effects.

Tony had heard about pharmaceutical cannabis therapy but was not convinced that it would be the right choice for him. Even with a prescription from his doctor, he was worried about the stigma: he didn't want his family to think that he was going to become a "hippie." He also learned that his health insurance didn't cover the cost of the medication, which was substantial.

I explained to Tony that my approach is to make this transition as non-threatening as possible. Because we knew that Epidiolex worked, I was able to start him on a regimen that was slightly higher than my lowest starting place. I explained that as his body becomes exposed to cannabis after a few days, his fat cells absorb some of the cannabinoids, and he would be able to have a durable, longer experience.

Tony called me a few weeks later. He let me know that the cannabis quickly ramped up in his system, and his seizures didn't last as long. By the third week, he was having fewer of them. What's more, the aftereffects of the seizures were also more tolerable. He also mentioned that his wife had noticed a dramatic change in his mood. He was less irritable and had a more positive overall outlook, making him much more pleasant to be around.

I was thrilled with his response, and told Tony that all of these signs pointed to the fact that he could increase his dose, and talk to his doctor about reducing the dosage of his anti-epileptic medications. I was hoping that this would prevent seizures from occurring completely, and asked him to come back after a few more weeks.

Within two months of his first visit with me, Tony was able to appropriately treat seizure strengths with a matching strength of cannabis. I taught him that there are going to be days when he could feel the seizure coming on, and in those instances, he can amp up that day as needed. He could keep something in a backpack for an emergency.

When It Comes to Seizures, Cannabis May Change Your Life

People with seizures often miss out on many of the parts of life that give us a sense of independence: full-time employment, travel far from home, driving a car without the fear of a sudden loss of control, or socializing without potentially embarrassing body movements. These scenarios, and sometimes more dire circumstances, occur because of the long recovery periods following seizures, including the temporary loss of cognitive functioning (brain fog), and the fear of not knowing when the next one will come on. The anxiety associated with missing out on what others consider "everyday life" can contribute to persistent undercurrents of depression and a reluctance to step outside of an already limited set of daily routines.

However, your life does not have to follow this script. Cannabis therapies are so effective in preventing seizures, and limiting their intensity and recovery time when they do occur, that they offer more than just good medicine. They provide the freedom to stop worrying about "what if" or "when," and give you back the power to live your life to its fullest potential.

Thousands of patients with seizures are discovering that pharmaceutical cannabinoid therapies are a simple option to help build a better life. As if reading from a common script, my epileptic patients tell me, on an almost daily basis, that these, as well as dispensary cannabis therapies, have saved their lives. In fact, the difference in their experience between their days before cannabis treatments and how they are living today is not subtle. They report that they feel empowered and confident, almost as if they are living a miracle, and they cannot imagine a life without cannabis to protect them.

CHAPTER 11

Physical Pain

Every day, I see patients who are struggling to manage their pain. For some, the pain is new, resulting from a recent injury. Others are experiencing chronic pain, such as joints that hurt. For a select few, their pain is all-consuming. And for many others, their pain is more manageable and comes and goes. My patients span a vast and varied range of pain: pain caused by muscular damage, inflammation, joint pressure (arthritis), or nerve problems. They sometimes know the source of their pain, but not always.

Regardless of the duration or the intensity, physical pain is profoundly disruptive of daily life. Pain can limit our physical capabilities, and it can be emotionally draining. Pain keeps many awake at night, so they are not getting the restorative sleep they need to help their bodies heal naturally. Constantly fatigued, many are frustrated with their work productivity and limited ability to socialize or function the way that they used to. Their pain becomes a part of who they are, a pervasive reminder that they aren't the person they used to be.

Many of my patients tell me that they have tried both over-the-counter pain relief options as well as the "big gun" prescription medications including opioids, with limited success. Many have put in their time with physical therapy, chiropractic, and home stretching. Some have even had unsuccessful surgeries, or their pain is a result of a surgery or treatment for another health issue, like cancer.

As you'll learn, when it comes to treating pain, no matter the source, guided cannabis therapy offers a significant answer. With one medicine, cannabis can address both the physical pain and the emotional burden. That's one of the biggest benefits about cannabis: it is not one pill for one ill. Instead, it's smoothing the entire system, addressing all the issues at the same time.

Cannabis can reduce pain whether it is localized, regional, or systemic. And the relief it provides does not leave you feeling sedated, so that you can go on and live the life you want without suffering. Best of all, my patients find the relief they are looking for. Again and again, I get the same types of feedback: *"I never thought I'd find something that would work for me," "When I take cannabis for a few days, I feel so much better,"* and *"I thought I had tried everything. I had no idea cannabis could work that way."*

Defining Pain

+ Local pain: my wrist hurts
+ Regional pain: my back hurts
+ Systemic pain: my whole body feels achy
+ Psychologically induced pain: pain created by stress or depression—i.e., clenched teeth/jaw pain, upset stomach, or malaise (lack of spirit) through the day
+ Acute pain: new, short-term pain resulting from an accident, fall, or injury
+ Chronic pain: ongoing, pervasive pain
+ Intermittent pain: pain that comes and goes—i.e., menstrual cramps or toothache

How Cannabis Addresses Pain

Cannabis doesn't magically make pain vanish. However, cannabis can offer a host of different and effective ways to diminish pain. From what I see each day with my patients, cannabis appears to be a far superior, multilateral treatment that is more likely to be effective for a greater number of people.

Improves Mobility

Cannabinoids are known to relax muscle tissues,[1] improve blood flow by temporarily modulating heart rate and blood-vessel thickness,[2] and modify the electrical
signaling of sensation, pressure, and pain-sensing nerves throughout the body.[3]
These properties can effectively address pain associated with muscle tension and/
or poor circulation. For example, one of cannabis's best-publicized benefits is relaxing the spasticity of muscle tension for those who suffer from multiple sclerosis.[4]
For these patients, as well as others experiencing muscle tension, cannabis facilitates the relaxation of tense and painful limbs, increases mobility, reduces muscle
spasms, and dramatically reduces localized discomfort. Products can be taken on
a regularly scheduled regimen, on an as-needed basis, or both.

Used preventatively, cannabis can help make exercise and physical therapy
more effective and more tolerable, in a similar way that stretching/warming up
gets the body ready for physical activity. Muscles are loosened, which lowers the
risk of injury. At the same time, when you are free from muscle pain, you can push
yourself past your usual limits. And with a more positive outlook, you will be more
likely to commit to your exercise program, and enjoy it.

Reduces Inflammation

Some types of pain are caused by the body's immune system reacting (or overre-
acting) to an injury or insult. When the reaction is appropriate, the area is flooded
with immune cells of various types in an attempt to protect injured organs and
parts, heal damaged tissues, repair broken connections, prevent infection or wound
contamination, and dispose of necessary waste products. That's why when you
hurt yourself, the area swells and becomes red: it is literally inflamed with helpful
molecules and critical elements of protection and signaling. However, sometimes
the inflammatory response goes overboard, and excess swelling causes additional
pain. Real damage is caused when the immune cells mistakenly attack the body's
healthy tissue. Before the advent of modern medicines, the innate immune system
response was the body's best and only line of defense against injury: the pain
caused by inflammation limited one's ability to put themselves in further danger.

In modern times, with modern medicines, the body's preprogrammed, and often extreme, inflammatory reaction is not necessary for survival, as pain is no longer a useful signal to remind the brain of your physical limitations. In essence, pain isn't required to prevent further injury.

One of the functions of the endocannabinoid system is to tamp down the inflammatory response. Cannabis has a direct effect on inflammation of all types, from acute to chronic, localized to systemic.[5] For example, pain caused by tissue or nerve damage responds well to cannabis's strong anti-inflammatory action. Even as it works to lower inflammation in one region, there is a positive down-stream benefit that incrementally reduces systemic inflammation: the cannabis lotion you apply to an arthritic knee is going to combat the inflammation at your knee, and as it gradually enters your bloodstream, you may also notice that you feel fewer symptoms of stress. The converse is also true: for those who use canna-binoid therapies as a system-wide anti-inflammatory to treat autoimmune condi-tions, they also find that their acutely inflamed tissues, such as acne, may improve. What's more, excessive swelling, which might sometimes shield damaged tissues from further insult, can also unnecessarily delay healing. In the presence of a strong anti-inflammatory medicine like cannabis, extraneous immune elements dissipate while more essential repair elements remain, and a more appropriate response can begin.

Many of my patients who are athletes apply lotions to swollen or painful joints for rapid relief and can continue to play their sport with reduced pain. My senior patients with local pain often prefer an edible choice that brings lasting relief. Cannabis therapies can be tolerated by a wide range of people, including those with organ damage (whether due to aging or injury), kidney disease, liver disease, sensitive stomachs, or allergies or aversions to other analgesics.

Heals Damaged Tissues

Stem-cell therapies that aid in rapid cellular regeneration are among the up-and-coming revelations in medical care. Preliminary research suggests that cannabis may play an important role in its success. Our stem cells orchestrate the regenerative system of replacing old cells with new ones. These stem cells respond to chemical signals that recruit their activation. There is now evidence suggesting that the endocannabinoid system is one of the communication channels transmitting this call for cellular renewal.[6] What's more, there is evidence that stem cells are sensitive to both endocannabinoids as well as external sources of cannabinoid molecules.[7]

For people who suffer with pain that has not responded well to traditional treatments, alternatives may offer hope. In animal models, damaged and injured tissues that are associated with pain—resulting from a burn, a bruise, joint pain, muscle strain, or a skin infection—appear to heal more effectively when the animal has been exposed to cannabinoids. The study confirms that the animal's stem cell mechanism is activated by cannabinoids in such a way that their tissues are regenerating more efficiently.[8] In my clinic, many of my patients have reported these same results with both topical and systemic cannabinoid products, and I expect my findings to be validated through more rigorous human study. My patients tell me that their injured tissues respond quickly and favorably to regular applications of cannabinoids.

Reduces the Damage from Everyday Life

The body is in a state of constant flux: some days you are building tissue, and some days you are breaking down tissue, in order to adapt to your environment. For example, each time you lift more weight than you are used to, your muscles tear ever so slightly, and then rebuild even stronger. Pain is a signal of these changes happening. Sometimes, the signals from damaged nerves, receptors, or tissue misfire, which can lead to chronic pain.

The chemistry of tissue breakdown and inflammation can be excessive, which leads to a state of physical stress. The mechanism of these chemical signals works through the endocannabinoid system. When external cannabis is present, the stress response recedes, and you will feel less pain, less anxiety, and less depression.

Jo Cameron: The Woman Who Didn't Feel Pain

The power of the endocannabinoid system to provide a source of relief is perfectly exemplified with the story of Jo Cameron, a Scottish woman who was identified as having two genetic mutations that protect her from feeling pain or anxiety. The two are related, and coincidentally allow for her body to underproduce an enzyme that breaks down anandamide, one of the endocannabinoids. In fact, she has twice as much anandamide as she should.[9]

With more anandamide always available in her system, Jo isn't protected from injury: in fact, these mutations often work against her. There have been many instances when she has been severely injured yet hasn't experienced the appropriate pain response. However, her story helps us understand the role of the endocannabinoid system when it comes to pain management. From there, we can infer the real role cannabis products can have in addressing pain for the rest of us.

Provides a Mental Distraction from Pain

In addition to its action on direct physical sensations of pain, cannabis provides easy access to a powerful set of psychological tools that can enable you to change your desired focus and attention, and in some circumstances, allow you to distract completely from your pain. As cannabis flows through the bloodstream, your ability to attend to multiple stimuli and sensations at the same time is broadened. This experience gives you the opportunity, and choice, to focus your attention on whatever may be more appealing than the experience of your pain. Overall, this will make your pain seem less intense.

Unlike narcotic medications like opioids, which unreservedly counteract the very sensations of pain and replace them with an overall sense of gratification, cannabinoids act on the same opiate receptors, yet less powerfully. Rather than thoroughly numbing pain, the experience of discomfort is downgraded and generally felt to be less intense or less all consuming. In essence, the pain is still there, yet there is a new ability to cope with it.

The Four Facets of Pain

I divide the way we experience pain into four domains: the production and transmission of pain signals, the interpretation of the signaling in the brain, the way we form memories of and attention to the pain, and the sense of personal identity that evolves from the experience of chronic pain. Most pain management medications are typically formulated to address only some of these mechanisms: For instance, ibuprofen quiets the initial transmission of the pain signal from its source. Opiates attack the reception and interpretation of pain signals in the brain, and they can affect the memory of pain. Antidepressants and anti-anxiety medications like gabapentin, amitriptyline, or doxepin also address components of the brain's signaling circuitry, the memory of pain, and the component of identity that frequently accompanies longer-term discomfort, yet they do not appear to have a meaningful impact on the production or transmission of pain signals.

Only cannabis attacks all of these mechanisms at once. Cannabinoids will quiet the localized transmission of pain signals where it hurts, mitigate the brain's attention to these weaker signals, temporarily obscure the memory of pain, and allow the sufferer to positively adjust their relationship with pain so that it no longer defines them.

The Transmission of Pain Signaling from a Source

Pain typically begins with an electrical signal sent from nerve endings anywhere on the body that are sensitive to pressure, temperature, and pain. This signal is then carried by and through a series of sequential nerve channels to the spinal cord, which ultimately transmits the signal to the brain for processing. Along this long pathway, physical gateways exist within the nerve cell walls, which can open and close, modifying the flow of the signal. When the gateway is closed, there is less signaling from the source, and you are less likely to notice local or regional discomfort. Cannabinoids can bind to these gateways, forcing them to open or close, thereby influencing the transmission of pain signals.[10]

Cannabis can also inhibit a nerve signal from moving forward by chemically limiting the preceding nerve from propagating a signal to the next. This dissipating nerve activity is referred to as *feedback inhibition*, and the result is that the initial pain signal will be diminished. This mechanism is why people describe the pain relief from cannabis as if someone has turned the volume down on their pain, rather than experiencing numbing or a blockage of sensation. This role for cannabinoids is part of every nerve communication in the body, which is why it is so effective on both local and systemic levels.

Damaged nerves may be sending pain signals, or they can send the wrong signals, which in and of themselves may be a source of pain. The nerves that misfire or miscommunicate are amenable to adjustment from outside sources. Just as ice can soothe damaged nerves, cannabis can effectively address the same issue, for longer periods of time. Many of my athletic patients use topicals to address pain caused by damaged nerves for its quick effects and easy access.

The Brain's Interpretation of Pain

Pain can occur anywhere in the body, but you do not fully experience the pain until the message gets to your brain. Cannabinoids may play a vital role in the brain's interpretation of these signals. When cannabinoids flow abundantly in the bloodstream, the brain receives a filtered message about the pain, even if the thousands of nerves in your hand are all sending the same pain signals. This occurs because the cannabinoids are affecting the nerve signals from the source, as well as in the brain. Increased cannabinoid signaling at nerve endings recalibrates the strength of the pain message to the brain.

When there is a filtered signal, you will be able to focus more on other stimuli rather than your pain. This is a powerful tool that can be modified by your personal preferences. Products that are high in THC seem to have a greater influence on the nerve signaling in the brain; products that are high in CBD seem to be more effective at quieting the nerve signaling coming from the body. What's more, the way your brain perceives and processes pain is also affected by the concept of set and setting. If your environment is soothing, you are more inclined to pay attention to it rather than your pain, because it is more pleasing. On the other hand, if your set and setting is consistently neutral or uncomfortable, you are more likely to focus on the pain signals, and cannabis won't bring about the results you are looking for.

In the brain, as well as throughout the body, cannabinoids encourage the creation of new cells and help to maintain their activation.[11] One of the ways we know this occurs is when we place someone who has taken cannabis into a functional MRI machine: the images light up with many activated regions throughout the brain. In this way, the hippies of the 1960s were right: cannabis is literally mind expanding. Another benefit of increased cell activation is that the percentage of cells transmitting pain signals is dwarfed in relation to the increase in overall activated nerves, resulting in a less overwhelming experience of pain.

The Memory of Pain

If you are someone dealing with chronic pain, wouldn't it be nice to have a vacation from time to time where you didn't have to think about it? If you are not experiencing the pain, that's one way to take a break. If you are not remembering that you are feeling pain, that's another way. Using memory as a way to reframe discomfort can be miraculously effective and is a completely new approach compared to traditional medical therapies. Through its ability to broaden your focus and escape from unpleasant thoughts and experiences, cannabis is a godsend for many people suffering from chronic pain.

Post-traumatic stress disorder (PTSD) is the extreme example. PTSD is the persistent recall of traumatic memories, especially memories related to physical pain. And as you learned, cannabis is an effective treatment for PTSD. Cannabis can also help you reframe your memories of traumatic pain. While you can't force yourself to forget something, cannabis primes memory nerves to signal less powerfully, and your attention can be drawn to many of the other competing signals. By lowering the volume of pain signaling, and expanding your focus to other stimuli besides pain, the memory of your pain will be reduced.

For example, treating pain with THC-dominant cannabinoids after a traumatic fall not only changes the signaling of the pain and lowers the inflammation, it might also help you focus on healing instead of worrying about the potential of falling in the future.

The Identity of Pain

The greater the struggle with pain, or the longer pain persists, the more likely one is to identify as a person whose life is oriented around their pain. When someone has consistently lost the fight against pain for years, it is logical for them to assume that they will always be in pain. The acceptance of this reality comes with a heavy expectation of chronic pain, the consistent stress of managing it, and the lifestyle and personality shifts that are strongly influenced by the limitations of endless pain.

Modern psychology offers some tools to engage with this phenomenon, including psychoanalytic therapy, cognitive behavioral therapy, and pharmacotherapy, which offers a chance to change your perspective, mood, and thought processes. Yet the rates of success of any of these therapies are limited. Cannabis therapy offers a different approach that is both well tolerated and appears to be much more effective. These treatments reduce pain at its origin, and they can help the reframe of self to pain through the signaling and memory mechanisms discussed above. With less pain and a reduced imprinting of memory, we can begin to see ourselves as more than just our pain.

MEET BOB AND LAURA

When I met Bob in 2021, he was sixty-six and described himself as "an old pothead" who had a stroke about five years earlier. Bob's stroke left him with weakness and lack of motion on his right side, which is his dominant side. He was confined to a wheelchair and told me that he was in constant pain. He was also having vascular issues related to his decreased circulation.

His wife and primary caregiver, Laura, is an occupational therapist working at a local hospital in Boston, and she'd attended an information session at work where they discussed the use of cannabis for pain control. After the conference, Laura sought my advice. They were using a pain management doctor in the same building where my office is, and that doctor recommended that they see me, as he's a big supporter of cannabis medicine.

Finding that pain management specialist was Bob's first piece of good luck, because prior to meeting him, they had tried to get an appointment with various pain management specialists, but most of them refused to treat Bob because he smoked marijuana, and they were intending to prescribe opioids. Laura told me that Bob had tried everything in terms of pain management, but nothing was really making a difference. He agreed to stop smoking so that he could take the OxyContin, and he was already taking gabapentin and nortriptyline. However, he would become very anxious when he couldn't have marijuana, and he found that when he was more anxious, he also had more pain.

I told Bob and Laura that I would be happy to work with his new pain management specialist to come up with a plan that included cannabis. I recommended that he look into pain patches, sold at the medical dispensary, that contained both THC and CBD, and he found some relief. Topical creams didn't seem effective; he tried sublingual tablets and tinctures but lack of oral motor skills from the stroke made them difficult to use and ineffective. The best intake turned out to be smoking.

The effects were literally immediate. Bob told me, "Before using cannabis, I lay in bed for practically four and a half years and I didn't improve in the least. I had been doing the exercises and everything. Then I started using the cannabis products. I went to bed one night feeling like my normal limited self, and I woke up the very next morning and started to notice a difference. It's been a steady, incremental improvement ever since, and in the last three months, I've improved tremendously. Now I can do more exercise. My right arm has a lot more mobility. My leg doesn't have nearly as much pain. I stopped taking the nortriptyline every day, I'm taking less of the gabapentin, and I'm taking hardly any of the Oxy. I still can't believe that the difference was overnight."

I was thrilled for Bob and Laura, but I was concerned that his results were not going to be replicable, since the flower products at dispensaries are often inconsistent, and smoking carries the risk of product mutation due to the excessive heat of combustion. Laura was excited to tell me that she understood my concern, but she had developed a method that was extremely replicable. She learned about certain terpenes that might be better suited for Bob's particular needs. So when she goes to the dispensary, she has a shopping list. "Instead of buying just based on THC percentages, we now look at the strains based on their terpenes. I choose the strains that have the terpenes that are directly related to his issues. I'm picking the terpenes that help with anxiety, that help with pain, that help with circulation. Then I actually mix different strains to create my own formulation for Bob. I'll mix the different flowers, I'll grind it, and then roll the joints with my handy-dandy little joint roller, which actually gets me the same measured dose because of how I pack it. This way I can replicate his treatment so that it's the same every day. And because it's so precise, we're buying less, not more. Bob used to smoke an ounce a week just for recreation. Now he's down to probably less than half that amount."

I was thrilled for the two of them, especially when I learned that adding cannabis to Bob's plan made caring for him easier. Laura told me, "The other painkillers were dampening his brain, whereas now his thinking is much clearer. He can now open containers and he's starting to use his hand to grasp utensils. He's moving around with more ease. He's got more strength. He's moving around better on the bed and on the couch where it takes less effort from me to care for him because he's able to roll himself in different positions. He's more independent in every way."

How Cannabis Compares to Other Pain Treatments

Cannabinoids can provide both short- and long-term pain relief in far different ways than many types of traditional medicines.

Over-the-Counter (OTC) Analgesics

Pain relievers like aspirin, acetaminophen (Tylenol), ibuprofen (Advil, Motrin), and naproxen (Aleve) are typically less effective than cannabis therapies. When you take these medications every day, you're really getting bursts of four- to six-hour relief, which when strung together through consistent, regular dosing, can feel like your pain is covered for the day, but you're really just getting incremental relief. Because cannabinoids are fat-soluble, and at least 10 percent of our body is comprised of fat cells, with consistent use, cannabinoids are stored in these and periodically released, even when you are not taking them. This provides for a slightly increased dose and longer-lasting coverage. What's more, the duration of action for cannabis products taken orally, particularly when taken on a schedule where you are taking more right before your pain returns, is much more powerful than shorter-acting agents.

And while they are effective, the OTC oral medications are known to have long-term side effects that are tied to regular use, including stomach irritation and blood clotting, and they can damage already weakened organs, like the kidneys and liver. And they are not known to impact your memory pain, or your sense of identity in terms of that pain, in a meaningful way.

Cannabinoids—CBD products in particular—can have the same short-term action without the withdrawal rebound. They act on the sensation and transmission of pain and inflammatory signals in the same way as most OTC pain relievers. Cannabis can also amplify the effects of these medicines, and the end result provides even more relief than either can individually. Over time, my patients end up using less over-the-counter remedies to treat their pain.

The anti-inflammatory properties of OTC pain relievers may also have potential psychological benefits similar to cannabis. For instance, preliminary studies have outlined the ability of anti-inflammatory agents such as ibuprofen and aspirin to safely curb symptoms of depression.[12]

Over-the-counter topicals can work in a variety of ways. Some work as numbing agents (Bengay, Biofreeze, Aspercreme, Icy Hot); others are anti-inflammatories (Voltaren); and some are antibacterial (Penetrex or Neosporin). Cannabis topicals are not numbing per se, but have effects to dial back the sensitivity of discomfort, and they are powerful anti-inflammatories. They also have antibiotic, antimicrobial, and antifungal properties.

Narcotics and Opioids

Narcotics are some of the most powerful pain relievers available, and they are prescribed by healthcare providers with great caution due to their addictive properties. They are typically used to treat moderate to severe acute or chronic pain and are often prescribed following surgery, injury, or cancer treatments. The complete class of narcotics include:

+ Codeine
+ Fentanyl
+ Hydrocodone
+ Hydromorphone
+ Meperidine
+ Morphine
+ Oxycodone
+ Tramadol

Not all narcotics are derived from the opium plant, though many are. Opioids like oxycodone are perhaps the best known and act as powerful anti-inflammatories that can work both locally as well as systemically.[13] However, they are highly addictive. When opiate receptors are saturated with opiate medicines, the receptors become overstimulated. In short time, the receptors instinctively recede in response to the excessive stimulation, so fewer receptors are present to match the incoming medicine. This causes a new, less comfortable equilibrium. Gradually, reduced receptor matching promotes new receptors to surface to accept the incoming medicine, and the cycle of ebbs and flows of pain continues. This is a phenomenon experienced by many who experience severe pain, as well as the millions addicted to opiates, as they struggle to outmaneuver the receptor-opiate balance with increasingly higher doses of medicine.

Not only are they highly addictive, opioids and other narcotics have a wide range of debilitating side effects, including constipation, nausea, fatigue, confusion, depression, reduced sex drive, and an overall increased sensitivity to pain. They can dull the mind as they ease the body. Worse, the body naturally builds tolerance to them, despite the persistence of pain. Gradually, more and more medicine must be taken to sustain relief, which is how addiction develops.

Cannabis can be a much more tolerable therapy with less intense side effects and risks compared to opioids. Cannabinoids activate the same receptors of the brain and the body that respond to opiates.[14] And because cannabis can hit the same receptors, it can help people who are addicted to opiates feel less uncomfortable, serving as an ideal tapering option.

When you build up your reservoir of cannabinoids, you will be able to achieve sustained relief and be better able to withstand the ebbs and flows of pain. What's more, my patients who are experienced cannabis consumers tend to require about 10 percent of the opiates prescribed after a surgery.

Injected Corticosteroids

Cortisone injections can help relieve pain by dramatically lowering inflammation in a specific area, most commonly treating different types of arthritis that affect your joints. They are also used to resolve back pain due to the injections' regional anti-inflammatory strength. While effective, these medications don't last forever, and quite often, only a limited number of injections will work. Research also suggests that these shots can damage the cartilage within a joint and nearby bones, and cause nerve damage if done incorrectly.

Cannabis is a powerful anti-inflammatory, and while it doesn't have the "one and done" effect of a steroid injection, it is a much safer treatment even if you have to use it regularly.

Cannabis Regimens for Pain

Cannabis therapies can be used among the first steps of treating acute pain, and they can continue to be used regularly if you suffer from chronic pain. As there are so many different permutations of pain, the following are broad recommendations.

Very few aspects of health are as much of a matched challenge of the psychological and physical as living life with pain. Chronic pain is multifaceted, often increases over time, and almost never goes away instantly, no matter the therapy. When one facet of the pain is treated, the disturbance in the other aspects related to the pain (inflammation, tissue damage, mood, unconscious compensation adaptations) can continue to be uncomfortable, and it may even be temporarily more uncomfortable until it has been appropriately treated.

Please try to be patient when you are treating pain, especially chronic pain. Be realistic with expectations. You will be able to see small, incremental changes before you achieve a less painful equilibrium. Many of my patients report that it took a few months before their chronic pain was effectively managed. Success may also require dosage adjustments in terms of strength and frequency. However, sticking with the program, close to 80 percent of my patients achieve the results they are looking for.

As they say, go low and slow. Cannabinoids slowly accumulate in your fat cells, and even the smallest doses will ease pain. Do not try a higher dose until you've gone a week or more without getting any relief. The greatest pitfall is taking too much at any given time, because the temporary discomfort of having excessive cannabis in your system can turn you off from the treatment entirely.

Local Pain:

+ **Onset timing:** Rapid onset (5–20 minutes).
+ **Short-acting versus longer-lasting:** Short-acting.
+ **Daytime or nighttime:** Can be applied both.
+ **Euphoric/non-euphoric:** Only rarely do topicals cause intense euphoria, even when they are high in THC.
+ **Product recommendation:** Topical administration (balms, patches).

Regional Pain:

+ **Onset timing:** Rapid onset (5–20 minutes).
+ **Short-acting versus longer-lasting:** Short-acting.
+ **Daytime or nighttime:** Can be applied both.
+ **Euphoric/non-euphoric:** Only rarely do topicals cause intense euphoria, even when they are high in THC.
+ **Product recommendation:** Topical administration (bath products, balms, patches).

Systemic Pain:

+ **Onset timing:** Delayed onset (at least an hour following oral therapies, longer if taken with food).
+ **Short-acting versus longer-lasting:** Long-lasting.

+ **Daytime or nighttime:** Can be applied both.
+ **Euphoric/non-euphoric:** Choose based on your personal preference at the moment; CBD and THC products are both effective.
+ **Product recommendation:** Oral administration, patches.

Psychologically Induced Pain:

+ **Onset timing:** Fast acting, microdosing.
+ **Short-acting versus longer-lasting:** Tinctures, inhalants (short-acting), edibles (long-lasting) taken together to provide comprehensive control and coverage.
+ **Daytime or nighttime:** Both. You can choose products with less THC for daytime use.
+ **Euphoric/non-euphoric:** Choose THC products.
+ **Product recommendation:** Tinctures, inhalants (short-acting), edibles (long-lasting).

Acute Pain:

+ **Onset timing:** Quick onset.
+ **Short-acting versus longer-lasting:** Short-acting.
+ **Daytime or nighttime:** Daytime.
+ **Euphoric/non-euphoric:** Choose based on your personal preference at the moment; CBD and THC products are both effective.
+ **Product recommendation:** Sublingual tinctures, topicals, suppositories, inhalants.

Chronic Pain:

+ **Onset timing:** Slow onset unless microdosing.
+ **Short-acting versus longer-lasting:** Longer-lasting.
+ **Daytime or nighttime:** Both.
+ **Euphoric/non-euphoric:** Choose based on your personal preference at the moment; CBD and THC products are both effective.
+ **Product recommendations:** Edibles, inhalants, patches.

Intermittent Pain:

+ **Onset timing:** Quick onset.
+ **Short-acting versus longer-lasting:** Short-acting.

+ **Daytime or nighttime:** Daytime.
+ **Euphoric/non-euphoric:** Choose based on your personal preference at the moment; CBD and THC products are both effective.
+ **Product recommendation:** Sublingual tincture, topicals, suppositories.

Product Recommendation: Topicals

If you are suffering from a specific pain, try short-acting topicals applied directly to where your pain is coming from. Certain lotion formulations work better on the skin than others. For example, a lotion made with more oil and less water is less likely to evaporate and can remain fixed to the skin tissues to have a lasting effect. There are also spa products, like bath bombs, that I have found to be incredibly effective for muscle relaxation. I often recommend patches for more long-acting relief, as they can provide deeper penetration and less evaporation.

MEET JOY

My patient Joy, who is eighty-five, cannot stand up straight. Joy suffers from spinal stenosis and is chronically hunched over: it is her body's effort to relieve the pressure on her spinal column. She came to see me because she was in constant pain, which was preventing her from doing the exercises that would make her frame-supporting musculature stronger. She also complained that she was not sleeping well.

I explained that cannabis treatment was not going to make the spinal stenosis go away, but it is going to make her more likely to succeed at physical therapy because she would be able to get some of her mobility back. Joy was skeptical at best. She had already been to an orthopedist who told her that the only recourse was going to be surgery, and she was really afraid of that option at her age. However, she couldn't continue living this way.

When we talked about treatment options, I realized immediately that Joy was not interested in feeling euphoric; she just wanted the pain to go away. We decided that she would start with a tincture and a lotion that her daughter could apply on her back. The tincture needed to come from a dispensary because I wanted her to have a CBD product during the daytime that also included a tiny amount of THC. The CBD-dominant mixture was sufficient to prevent the euphoric effects from THC, which might have interfered with Joy's desired state of mind, and offered a high dose of anti-inflammatory compounds. I suggested that she take an edible at night that was higher in THC so that she could sleep better, and the euphoric effect wouldn't bleed into her daytime activities.

About three or four days after she came to see me, Joy called me on the phone. She was elated because she was already sleeping better, and she wanted to know if there was anything stronger that she could try for her pain. She agreed to try a higher-dose CBD chocolate bar. Two weeks later she called again to tell me that she was ready to go back to the physical therapist. She was sleeping really well and her mood was elevated because she was more comfortable during the daytime.

I've been seeing Joy every six months for the past three years. She's been doing her physical therapy regularly and seeing results. She's not standing perfectly straight, but she can make it from the supermarket to her car without feeling unsteady. She can carry her groceries from the car into her home. She's functional in a way that she hasn't been in years. She can now do everything she wants to do, albeit in a little bit of discomfort, which she is not really bothered by because of the cannabis.

This story does have a happy ending, but it's also a cautionary tale. When I saw Joy last, she told me that she had been in the hospital because she had taken a fall. While there, the testing picked up that she had a urinary tract infection. The problem was that Joy didn't feel the typical pain associated with it.

I explained to Joy that she needed to dial back her cannabis dosage so that she could be in better touch with her body. Pain is a natural, adaptive signal that informs us when something is wrong. If you tune down that message, you risk harming yourself. In this case, Joy could have become septic because of the infection, and it might have led to death. We decided that she would take three or four days off from her cannabis protocol every month, so that she could check in with her body.

CHAPTER 12

Gastrological Issues

Gastrointestinal (GI) complaints are among the most common of the adult illnesses, and also some of the most challenging to treat effectively. The range of symptoms and conditions is vast, and each person has a different tolerance to discomfort: what might be mildly upsetting for one is "excruciating" for another. And like other forms of physical pain, an episode can be acute, chronic, or intermittent, and discomfort can be felt locally, regionally, or systemically. These disparate issues can be caused by a foreign invader like bacteria, or can be connected to the stresses of a job or relationship, or a response to something you ate or drank. What's more, gastrointestinal issues are exhausting to deal with and can affect our outlook on life.

Guided cannabis treatments are thought to address the root causes of many stomach issues, like inflammation, infections, and the effects of stress and anxiety. Cannabis can also relieve the symptoms of abdominal discomfort. At present, there is only a smattering of scientific research that shows strong correlations between cannabis therapies and their effectiveness on gastrointestinal issues. However, my patients would say differently. Every day, they are proving that the theoretical is a reality: they are managing their symptoms and consistently finding real relief with cannabis, when other, more conventional treatments have failed them or come with intolerable side effects.

While the precise mechanisms of the effects of cannabis on the gastrointestinal system are still a source of intense ongoing investigation, we do know that the gastrointestinal tract is rich in cannabinoid receptors.[1] What's more, cannabinoids, terpenes, and flavonoids act in the body synergistically. Not only do these compounds affect the action of one another,[2] they also help to balance the complex overlapping tides of chemical and nerve signaling within the gastrointestinal system. The result is a new equilibrium that facilitates healing and eases discomfort. My experience with patients has taught me that the common perception that THC or CBD alone is the magic answer is inaccurate when it comes to the gut.

You have already learned that there are direct effects of cannabinoids on nerves and inflammation, and on blood flow. And cannabis is used to soothe emotional distress. Each of these effects offers its own form of relief for gastrointestinal ailments, alone or in combination, depending on the underlying cause. For example, if your stomach distress is related to autoimmune issues, like colitis, the ability of cannabinoids to stimulate tissue healing and strong anti-inflammation is what helps to quash a flare-up of disease. The antimicrobial features of cannabis products appear to rebalance the gut flora toward a healthier equilibrium, aiding in the resolution of chronic bloating, diarrhea, constipation, and nauseousness. At the same time, cannabis can address the anxiety that comes with or, in many cases, may be causing the problem.

There is debate in the scientific community about the origins of common gastrointestinal illnesses. Some believe that they are attributable to modern habits or exposures, while others point to archeological evidence of autoimmunity that predates modern humans as a species altogether.[3] Whether or not foods and eating habits are the cause of GI illness, or the ultimate origin is more deeply rooted in genetics and evolution, effective treatments for bowel diseases seem to work best when they imitate nature, including natural foods and processes.

In nature, animals of all types eat a variety of plants, including flowers, fruits, berries, nuts, and vegetables, and some also eat other animals. Buried within these foods are nutrients, including proteins, fats, minerals, and vitamins, as well as other biologically active compounds that can help to protect against unhealthy exposures (UV light, chemical toxins, infectious agents, etc.). The very same compounds that may protect a plant from UV light damage can also protect whoever is eating that plant, by means of the very same molecular machinery. Through other mechanisms, some plant molecules can interact with the communication system of the body to hush the activity of the immune system. Through their experimenting with nature and the biological effects of certain plants, early humans learned of plants' medicinal qualities, which we later adapted to create the medicines we have today. For instance, salicylic acid, the active ingredient in aspirin, is readily found within the bark of the willow tree.[4]

Cannabis alone produces over six hundred compounds that are also found throughout nature. Its natural laboratory is vast, and there is still much yet to be discovered. The clinical reality, ahead of the knowledge to explain it, is showing that the compounds in cannabis are improving health with remarkable effectiveness.

You May Be Endocannabinoid Deficient

People who have had GI issues, or grapple with dysfunction, may be endocannabinoid deficient.[5] This term, first proposed in 2001, is meant to encourage more thoughtful consideration of the impact that the endocannabinoid system may have on everyday physiology. It is currently being used for illnesses like irritable bowel syndrome, where a psychosomatic label, as well as the failure of traditional therapeutic interventions, have left sufferers searching for answers to the cause of their problems. This deficiency may be the exact reason why cannabis products have been so effective, where other therapies have failed.

Using Cannabis to Treat GI Inflammation and Infection

The gastrointestinal tract is one of several essential "homes" for your immune system, where it can gather and share information and form offensive and defensive strategies for cellular protection. These homes include components of the skin, areas within nasal passages, the respiratory tract, the digestive tract, and others that host exceptionally high concentrations of immune-supportive inflammatory cells. Suppressing autoimmunity is one benefit of cannabis taken into the gastric-associated immune tissues. When cannabinoids activate these regions, they impact by correcting an inappropriately reacting immune system, improve the healing of damaged tissues, and provide a dramatic relief of discomfort. And when your immune system is balanced, you will be better able to suppress GI infections like diverticulitis and H. pylori when you are faced with them.

Conditions like irritable bowel syndrome (IBS), Crohn's disease, and ulcerative colitis occur when the immune system is not functioning correctly, and the body attacks its own cells. The result is an abundance of inflammation and tissue damage, both of which can cause physical discomfort and stress. As you've learned, cannabis can powerfully address inflammation and tissue damage, so that the region can heal on its own. It can also enhance stem cell production, providing another avenue of healing.

The typical medical treatment for those who have Crohn's disease or ulcerative colitis is high-dose steroids to treat symptom flares, but they do not cure the disease. Existing treatments can be effective yet are known to be debilitating. Some people with Crohn's disease have to take time off work due to their symptoms, pain, or the side effects of traditional medications. Newer, biologic medicines have also proven to be effective. Yet these come with their own set of side effects, including lowering one's overall immune response to other diseases.

Cannabis works in a similar way to both classes of medication but with fewer detrimental side effects. In a series of Israeli studies from 2017, patients with either Crohn's disease or ulcerative colitis showed great improvements using cannabis products.[6] While the exact mechanism was unclear, the positive results could be attributed to cannabis's ability to reduce both inflammation and overall anxiety levels. Cannabis is not curing the physiologic or inflammatory issues that are at the core of GI illnesses; it is merely addressing the symptoms.

However, cannabis therapies can help people get off these strong medicines or not need them as often. In 2021, the same group of researchers found that cannabis can reduce the number of flares, and when the flares occur, they can be better managed.[7] I have worked with many patients who have Crohn's disease and have weaned them off their biologics or steroidal treatments because they're getting the relief they need from cannabis.

Cannabis and the Microbiome

We also know that a mellow immune system is less likely to react to bacterial imbalances in the gut. Known collectively as a *microbiome*, these bacteria can be both helpful and harmful: some believe that a bacterial imbalance of too many bad bacteria is at the heart of many GI illnesses—and even overall health.[8]

Cannabinoids may have disruptive effects on the microbiome, and this mechanism may be another factor in how it heals the gut. We do know that CBD and THC have been studied in both low and high doses, and it's clear that high doses can have a powerful impact on bacteria in the microbiome. In high doses, it has been found to function as an antibiotic,[9] an antifungal,[10] and an antimicrobial.[11] The bacteria, fungi, and viruses that live in the gut all require very specific environments to replicate and thrive. Cannabis has properties that both stop the growth of, and can kill, these offenders and allow the growth of more beneficial bacteria.

Addressing Physiological GI Issues

Your entire GI tract operates on *peristalsis*, the sequential contraction of smooth muscle that moves foods through the phases of digestion. Some bowel illnesses are attributed to intestinal muscles misfiring or misfunctioning. Cannabis seems to reawaken effective communication in these muscular systems so that they can function better, yet we don't quite understand the mechanism of how it works. We do know that, generally, people who are consuming cannabis feel a normalization of bowel flow. Cannabis may be resetting these muscles to the way that they were designed to operate; if so, it would be the first medicine of its kind to do so.

The stomach also contains an incredibly dense area of nerves. Some bowel illnesses are attributed to the misfiring or over-/under-action of these nerve networks.

For instance, nauseousness is often caused by the mixed signaling of nerves: the brain may be receiving one type of auditory signal that doesn't match with a visual cue, causing dizziness. Or perhaps the visual cues are different from the orientation of the body in space, such as the nauseousness associated with motion sickness. Cannabis can soothe this type of upset stomach by dialing down the volume of nerve transmission. When cannabis is present, hyperactive nerves settle so that they can better regulate themselves to a healthy equilibrium.

The following chronic GI issues are disorders primarily related to mechanical flaws in the digestive tract:

+ **Constipation:** A temporary bout of constipation can be caused by food choices and inadequate hydration; a chronic condition can also be caused by illness in the gut or the inadequate forward movement and processing of food. For those who do not find relief with a daily dose of dietary fiber or increasing fluids in their diet, cannabinoids typically provide a surprising level of relief. Cannabinoids taken in oil formulations—such as tinctures and edibles—may relieve constipation just as taking mineral oil without cannabinoids acts as a laxative. In that sense, if someone's constipated, a substantial amount of the oil (1–2 tablespoons) can help loosen things up in the short term. In the long term, the systemic presence of cannabinoids appears to work effectively and reliably. The mechanisms are still being studied, but cannabinoids are thought to stimulate the parasympathetic nervous system, which is responsible for the forward movement in the gut, in the same way that the engine stimulates the forward movement of a car. Similarly, cannabinoids may be exerting a relaxation effect for those portions of the gut that may be tense or cramped, thus supporting increased forward movement of the gastrointestinal system and relieving some types of habitual constipation.

+ **Diverticulosis:** This disorder is an outpouching of one set of tissues protruding into another layer of tissue. It doesn't become diverticulitis until it comes into contact with bacteria and the body launches an immune response. This disorder can cause excruciating pain locally and regionally, and can be a source of anxiety related to the pain. Cannabis seems to address the pain, and it may prevent the area against infection by addressing inflammation. It may also prevent further structural damage, like abscesses and perforations in the colon as it helps to reset and promote the forward momentum of digestion.

+ **Fecal incontinence:** Fecal accidents are an embarrassing reality for those suffering from a host of physical issues that affect the musculature of sphincters, which enables controlled bowel flow. For some, the physical cause for this problem is difficult to identify, and they are treated for potential psychological origins. My patients who suffer from fecal incontinence report that cannabinoid treatments appear to be more effective than the absence of treatment. Cannabinoids may be relaxing stiff or spasmed musculature; they may be distracting the parts of the mind that are causing a loss of control; or perhaps they support healing of local tissue or functioning nerve connections that were believed lost to repair.

+ **Gas:** The origins of gas/bloating can be physical, environmental, or infectious. There are many foods that create gas, including nuts, legumes, foods high in fiber, and for some with food intolerances, the list goes on to include milk, gluten, eggs, protein, seafood, and others. The treatment of bloating and gas with cannabis is not a common practice even among medical cannabis clinics, and the mechanism of action is not yet known. Yet many patients I see have reported improvements with flatulence. This may well be due to the fact that when they are taking cannabis they are less bothered by their gas, or more distracted to notice its frequency, but the trend is still notable.

+ **Heartburn and gastroesophageal reflux disease (GERD):** These conditions are related to an overabundance of stomach acid. Reflux disease is often caused by a loose sphincter at the junction of the stomach and esophagus, so acid from the stomach, which is constantly churning, is getting tossed into the lower esophagus, spreading acid, which then damages esophageal tissues. For some, heartburn is related to bacterial origins, like H. pylori. For others, excessive acid may be environmental, created from stress or poor diet (too much food, or eating the wrong foods). Sometimes, excessive acid causes peptic ulcers, when there is too much acid in one place or not enough protection there, and the acid from the stomach eats into its lining, creating a crater of damage. Whatever the cause, the regular consumption of cannabinoids seems to be remarkably effective for chronic conditions, due to its antibacterial, stress-relieving, and appetite-regulatory effects. Together, these factors can de-escalate acid production. I have found that it also works for my patients as needed for intermittent bouts of acid sensitivity.

+ **Vomiting:** Vomiting is a reflex that evacuates the stomach in cases of anxiety (as in eating disorders such as anorexia or bulimia) or the ingestion of a disagreeable food or toxin. The explosive tension is a resetting to the nervous system associated with the gut and the musculature to which it is directly connected. For those who suffer from chronic vomiting, this reflex is providing relief but occurring too frequently. Cannabis can insert a relaxation stage, which either resets the system or allows healing to take place that would not otherwise occur.

Cannabis Can Increase or Decrease Appetite

Overeating and undereating are complex issues related to healthy functioning of the body, stable functioning of the mind, and effective internal communication between the brain and the gut. The endocannabinoid system is pivotal to all three processes. What's more, it is the very substance of appetite. When cannabinoid receptors are activated, they provide the essential status signaling that tells us when we are hungry, or when we are satisfied. When someone doesn't want to eat, THC products will help them create a ravenous appetite. When someone is overeating, the presence of CBD-dominant products helps them feel satiated sooner. Cannabinoids like THCV (derived from THC and not CBD) are also associated with effective appetite suppression.

Some illnesses—including constipation, diarrhea, nauseousness, reflux disease, and ulcers—are related to overeating or poor diet habits. Oftentimes, people don't eat healthy foods, and when they eat too much, it's usually unhealthy food that they overeat. If cannabis can pull back their desire to eat, there's a benefit. Conversely, there are many illnesses that reduce appetite, including cancer, anxiety, depression, and chronic pain, where cannabis can help both the illness itself and improve appetite.

I have also found that my patients are more likely to adhere to the necessary changes in diet when they are also consuming cannabis. When someone is trying to follow a strict diet, whether it's to lose weight, gain weight, or to maintain a healthier digestive system, they're often picking foods toward their specific aims, which may not be as pleasurable as the chocolate cake they are giving up. Our brains are hardwired to seek pleasurable experiences, which is one reason why it's very easy to be thrown off course when you are confronted with foods that taste nice. For example, someone who has celiac disease has to avoid gluten, and sometimes the choices are limited and boring. Yet when there is cannabis present, you can focus on your higher priority and enjoy the foods that may be less than tasty because it allows for a greater sensory experience. You can focus on the chewiness, on the crunchiness, or on the saltiness. So when my patients ask me for a tip to help them succeed with their diet, I often tell them to take a cannabis product before making an eating decision. Just a small dose will give you an extra level of command over your own body and your own desires.

One caveat to remember is that THC products will likely make you feel hungry. This occurs because cannabis stimulates hunger centers in the brain and gut, and it dries out the body, including the mouth and throat. These are both powerful natural signals to eat and drink. This effect can be countered with CBD products. And by anticipating these effects, you can make healthy choices when you are hungry.

The Relationship Between Mental Distress and Stomach Upset

When you are experiencing anxiety or stress, your stomach produces acid, your heart races, and the stress hormone cortisol floods the body, preparing the body to take action against imminent danger. This danger can be real, anticipated, or imagined. It is partly for this reason that any form of stress can be so dangerous. Many of my patients are stressed about eating because they know they won't feel well afterward, or they are worried about their weight, or they are concerned about feeling too much pleasure from food itself.

The stress response creates cycles of energy expenditure that are unhealthy and lead to weight gain, the failure of effective digestion and absorption of nutrients, and faulty signaling from the gut to the rest of the body. The presence of increased acid alone causes physical damage to the whole GI tract, including the stomach, esophagus, intestines, and so on.

This is the mechanism that connects mental distress with the physical manifestation of GI issues. But we also know that people who suffer from GI issues often experience tremendous mental anguish related to how they feel about themselves and their condition. These two elements create a vicious cycle that damages the body even further. One can try to fix the systemic stress through therapy, meditation, and medications. One can also try to fix their stomach issues with changes in diet, medications, or even surgery. Cannabinoids represent a third option that may be new for many people because they can reset both the brain and the gut.

We do know that cannabis products, especially those that are THC dominant, will make your daily experience calmer and less stressed. Those same products may help calm your stomach pains and digestive ailments that are caused by stress. The reason is that the stomach houses the same brain chemical receptors that the endocannabinoid system binds with; in essence you are treating the brain and the gut at the same time. Second, when someone is calm, the nerves that activate digestion and amplify calm in the body—the parasympathetic nervous system—promote the forward movement of digestion. And when there is increased digestive flow, the tissues in the gut are less obstructed and experience less pressure on any one area, facilitating better flow of nutrients, as well as creating space for healing damaged tissues.

Most importantly, cannabis opposes the action and release of cortisol and other stress hormones, ending the stress response.[12] Its mechanism is still under investigation but appears to be a stabilization of stress hormones so that they interrupt their own signaling pathways. In the short term, people feel amplified emotions. In the long run, they experience lasting calm and durable relaxation, and GI-system symptoms seem to vanish.

Further still, consuming cannabis products regularly also helps to ease the experience of suffering. With cannabinoids, the daily burden of my patients' gastric illnesses can be slowly separated from their sense of identity, at the same time as the body heals from the physical damage. By managing both the stress and the physical symptoms, my patients can disentangle their identity from their physical maladies.

A GI Case for CBG

Each cannabinoid works like a key that fits into certain locks. Some cannabinoids, like THC and CBD, can function as master keys because they fit into many different locks, and consequently, can address many health issues. Others may fit into multiple locks, but appear to unlock a particular door more easily. That's the case of CBG, which is in the CBD family, in that it is non-intoxicating, so it doesn't have any of the limitations that are commonly attributed to the euphoric effects of THC. In the available clinical studies, it seems that CBG has a particularly effective and soothing quality on a wide variety of GI tract illnesses.[13] CBG is quite easy to find: it's all over the internet. CBG drops are being added to a CBD product to make CBD plus CBG. One can buy CBG flower. One can buy CBG in a wide variety of formulations.

A regimen high in CBG seems to calm the stomach ecosystem toward a state of relaxation, reprieve, and balance. Patients with overactive acid production typically find themselves less acidic, and patients with chronic inflammation find themselves with fewer areas of inflammation and disrepair. I could have two patients walk in the door, and one has chronic constipation, and one has chronic diarrhea, and I can prescribe the same CBG treatment. In my experience, CBG products offer a slam-dunk cannabinoid for relief among patients who are suffering with severe bowel illnesses.

MEET AUSTIN

Austin is a patient of mine in his early thirties, and had been consuming cannabis products from his local dispensary for two months in an effort to treat his irritable bowel syndrome. He had heard that some of his friends had better success when they focused on CBG products, and he had recently read a blog post about the benefits. Austin called me because he wanted to know if I could help him fine-tune his regimen to provide consistent relief.

I agreed with his research. I explained that switching to CBG products wouldn't provide an overnight fix, but that, given his symptoms, I was confident that in four or five months, and with consistent use, he would likely feel much more stable and be in a strong position to reconsider his need for the traditional medicines he was also taking to control his IBS. I explained that GI issues revolve around an inflammatory cycle, so they may take a longer time to resolve, no matter what type of cannabinoid product is involved.

Austin took my advice. At his next appointment, four months later, he was beaming. He told me, "Dr. Caplan, you were right. I'm so much more comfortable and I haven't needed most of my other medicines anymore. This CBG is working fantastically."

I was thrilled to hear about Austin's success, and we discussed the importance of staying the course with CBG at a maintenance dosage, even if his symptoms of IBS were so strongly improved.

Just Because We're Talking About Gut Health Doesn't Mean You Have to Choose Oral Products

The true purpose of the stomach is to destroy whatever comes into the body, including foods and medications. In reality, far fewer amounts of any medication, including cannabinoids, are getting to where you want when you eat them: they are being destroyed by the acid and churning in the stomach on the way. In essence, very little of the medicine that you took is really addressing your complaint, either because it is difficult to absorb, the absorption process is impaired, or the medicine itself is being digested.

The exceptions to this rule are cannabis edibles that are high in fats or oils, which offer an energy-dense product of high value to the body. A special transport molecule, called the *chylomicron*, protects dietary fats and oils from acidic destruction in the stomach, which gives oily products that might otherwise evade effective absorption the opportunity for rapid and efficient entry into the bloodstream. By adding cannabis products to fats and oils, you will be able to access more of them.

Another choice that is less affected by digestion is rectal suppositories. These products are directly absorbed into the bloodstream, and they can be used for those who suffer from hemorrhoids in the same way one would use Preparation H. For those who have a damaged digestive tract and cannot, or don't want to, use inhalation for systemic absorption, suppositories are an effective alternative. I have helped many families with a loved one who cannot eat or take medications either orally or by inhalation, for whom suppositories have made a remarkable difference. For instance, patients under intensive care in the hospital may not be able to take cannabinoids by mouth or inhalation, but suppositories provide an effective, simple alternative.

Topicals can also be applied to the abdomen, directly where you may be experiencing a particular pain, even though the origin of the pain may be far deeper.

Regimens for GI Illnesses

Some of the traditional medications that treat GI issues have a toxic profile, and while they provide symptom relief, they cause greater health problems elsewhere. One example is proton pump inhibitors (PPIs) such as omeprazole. These medications successfully treat GERD yet are addictive and linked to osteoporosis and kidney disease. In contrast, cannabis does not seem to cause other damage in the body or brain. It's so safe that my patients are excited to try it, and then impressed when they see how much better they are feeling.

Cannabis treatments are equally appropriate for severe GI illnesses as well as acute pains and digestive discomforts. However, the cannabis prescription for GI issues can get somewhat specific. As you've learned, CBG/CBD/CBC seem to be better at addressing stomach concerns, including intestinal inflammation.

On the other hand, THC is better at fighting nauseousness. THC, Delta-8, or CBN are better at appetite stimulation, while THC-V and CBD are better at appetite suppression.

+ **Onset timing:** For an acute discomfort, you can use a high dose of fast-acting cannabis product, and you're going to distract yourself nicely from feelings of pain. For treating chronic illnesses, you need to be medicating regularly, and fast-acting isn't always required.

+ **Short-acting versus longer-lasting:** Serious medical concerns, like chronic GI issues, are amenable to long-term consumption of consistent doses. You may find that you will not require high doses provided that you maintain a consistent regimen that creates a systemic load of cannabinoids. Certain organs around the GI tract are less likely to receive the necessary therapeutic volume of cannabinoids without a steady amount available.

+ **Daytime or nighttime:** It doesn't really matter when you take CBD/CBG as long as there is consistency in timing and dosage, especially if you are treating a chronic stomach problem.

+ **Euphoric/non-euphoric:** Non-euphoric options, which are often taken in too-small dosages, seem to manage issues associated with inflammation effectively, but the low doses frequently are inadequate to effectively manage the emotional symptoms that are connected with GI illnesses, such as the depression or anxiety. When taking non-euphoric, CBD-dominant products, you may require higher dosages. When taking euphoric, THC-dominant options, or combinations of the two, you will likely find lower dosages to be just as effective.

+ **Product recommendation—CBG:** CBG can be a dominant part of a GI treatment plan. It should be used as a component of any regimen, even when you are focusing on THC-dominant products.

+ **Cannabis and medications:** Typically, my patients add cannabis to their existing GI medication routine. Over time, they slowly taper off the other medicines and increase their consumption of cannabis. Do not stop taking prescription medications without fully consulting your prescribing healthcare provider. You should feel comfortable with cannabis and how it might make you feel before you entertain reducing other medicines or getting off them.

Cannabis and Making Good Food Choices

While eating naturally is often the healthiest option, eating consistently unbalanced meals appears to be one of the strongest risk factors for gastrointestinal illnesses, including foods that are made with synthetic preservatives, foods taken in excessive quantities, or food that is loaded with too much of one ingredient (too much carbohydrate, too much protein, too much fat, etc.). You may have heard this before: choose a varied diet that includes lots of fresh vegetables, healthy proteins, limited added sugars and fats, and avoid processed foods. In reality, a varied diet is analogous to the cannabis plant itself, which naturally contains many of the exact same nutrients, vitamins, and minerals found in the healthiest food choices. If you are already making the best choice by treating yourself with a healthy option like cannabis, don't focus on foods that will derail your best efforts. Natural foods, grown from the earth, will amplify the benefits that cannabis is already providing.

Certain foods may very well be the cause of your discomfort. Your body grows from the ingredients you feed it. You can investigate which foods may be troublesome for you by trying an elimination diet while you are treating your symptoms. You may find that your favorite foods are the culprit, but as I tell my patients, taste is just one reason to pick foods. If you pay attention to more than your taste buds, you may find the relief you are looking for.

CHAPTER 13

Skin Conditions

To my mind, cannabis is the Swiss Army knife of skin care treatments, while all other skin medicines are individual knives. Traditional medicines that treat skin disorders, including both prescription and over-the-counter remedies, typically only act in one capacity: they can moisturize, reduce inflammation, or fight off offenders. Many of these skin treatments can dry out the skin as a side effect, which in most instances is the exact opposite of what patients require, as moisture supports the skin's natural physical barrier of defense against damage. Some ointment medications contain steroids to which people develop tolerances, and they can impact our DNA and other organs that may not be the target of therapy.

In contrast, cannabis therapies do not have these negative side effects. More importantly, the same treatment can address all of these issues, even at the same time. There's no question in my mind that cannabis is the most effective skin medicine, including steroids, antifungal medicines, and local pain relievers.

Your skin issues are as individual as you are and can occur in mind-bending, and often frustrating, combinations. Some are caused by the environment— poor diet, exposure to toxins, infections, or too much sun—while others are autoimmune in nature. Whether you are dealing with something that's mildly annoying or painful, cannabis can help.

The multi-therapeutic option can also activate the skin to look younger and healthier. A child's skin is supple, smooth, healthy, and repairs easily; these features may be directly related to the fact that children naturally have an enhanced endocannabinoid system, which gradually declines with age. So, when my patients ask me if cannabis is the fountain of youth, it's really hard to say no.

The following are just some of the conditions that my patients have reported using cannabis therapies for as treatment and have seen significant results:

+ Acne
+ Alopecia (hair loss)
+ Eczema
+ Fungus
+ Hyperpigmentation (dark circles under the eyes, for instance)
+ Neuropathy (shingles, pain)
+ Pruritis
+ Psoriasis
+ Raynaud's disease
+ Rosacea
+ Skin cancers
+ Sunburn
+ Sweating disorders
+ UV protectant (sunscreen)
+ Varicose veins
+ Vitiligo
+ Wound healing
+ Wound pain
+ Wrinkles

Cannabis: The Skin's Ultimate Reset Button

For all of these conditions, cannabis seems to function as a reset button for the skin. There is a thriving endocannabinoid hub that flourishes in the skin, which may be the reason why cannabis can be used to treat a wide variety of conditions. Cannabinoid receptors have been found in every level of skin cells, hair follicles, the oil-producing sebaceous glands, sweat glands, and even the deep stem cells that foster healing and growth of new generations of skin.[1] Whether you are dealing with wrinkles, varicose veins, or acne, every tissue that is exposed to cannabis topicals is capable of receiving this reset signal, even tissues far beneath the skin layers, including joints, muscles, and our body's internal organs.

The skin, like all organs in the body, is a complex organization of cells that send and receive molecular signals, either between skin cells or to other surrounding tissues. As you've learned, the molecules and receptors that make up the endocannabinoid system are part of the fundamental language of internal body communication, as well as part of the body's dynamic relationship to its environment. Skin issues occur as a result of both internal and external forces. When too little water is present, tissues become dehydrated. When there is a temporary swell in testosterone, the hormone stimulates excessive oil production. Yet when cannabinoids are present, they seem to reset the way that tissues receive or transmit signals, including how nerves may be transmitting signals and the way that skin cells receive signals to thrive or self-destruct.

To better understand how the endocannabinoid communication system might help so many different skin conditions at the same time, it's important to know that endocannabinoid tone is not merely a one-way on/off signal, but a combination of both activating and deactivating molecules and receptors. Some elements within the endocannabinoid system send very simple "turn on" signals, while other elements send "turn off" signals. Still others have more nuanced action, not quite activating or deactivating, but rather discouraging other molecules (perhaps stimulating, perhaps relaxing) from engaging at all.

When certain cells are switched on by particular cannabinoid receptor activation, tissues may interpret the receptor action as a signal to thrive and grow. Or, if those same cannabinoid receptors are switched off by an opposing cannabinoid signal, the same tissue may collapse and wither. For example, research in dental medicine has discovered that gum tissues can thrive and grow in abundance when exposed to one set of cannabinoids. Yet when the same oral tissues are stripped of those experimental cannabinoids or presented with cannabinoids that oppose the stimulating action of the first cannabinoids, the gum tissues appear to recede and decay.[2]

There are numerous conditions where the ability to mediate between signals of growth or death can affect your health and wellness. In conditions of skin overgrowth, excessive sweating, overactive oil glands, skin tags, skin cancers, tumors of deep tissues, excessive hair growth, or discolorations in the skin, topical cannabinoid formulations can be surprisingly effective in their ability to curb growth. And, in situations of insufficient growth, including hair loss, varicose veins, loss of pigment, rashes, excessive dry skin, and all manner of local wounds, certain cannabis formulations will also provide equally meaningful improvements. For this reason, cannabis is beginning to be known for its equalizing effect: it levels extremes using the same core product.

Through my patients' successes, cannabinoid therapies have taught me that the body seems to take what it needs from them, and it suffers no harm if there is an excess. Tissues that are already healthy seem to effectively ignore new cannabinoid signals that are curative (or destructive as the case may be), so that the medication focuses only on the afflicted tissues. This approach to therapy is unusual in medical treatment because it so closely mimics natural healing. Not only is cannabis a natural product, it activates your skin's inherent healing system, which promotes a balanced response of both repair and disruption. Ideally, finding a product that offers true full-spectrum cannabinoids, including CBD, THC, terpenoid, and flavonoid elements, is the way to achieve best results. We also know that isolated distillates of cannabis, including oily forms of nearly purified THC or pure CBD, provide a less effective treatment.

While a localized approach may seem to be offering a temporary fix, cannabis therapies seem to be normalizing a wider region of body tissue beyond the area of application, and for an extended period of time. By doing so, cannabis may be functioning as an anti-inflammatory, antibacterial, antifungal, and antiviral treatment, all at the same time.

Experiment Until You Get the Desired Result

The surprising benefits of cannabis therapies, seemingly across so many different skin conditions, have garnered both intense optimism and skepticism. You may be among those who have heard from friends or family the miraculous benefits from cannabis skin products. At the same time, there are just as many anecdotes where cannabinoids were tried and failed to produce a positive effect. These ambiguous reports are confusing and, for many, frustrating.

My suggestion is simple: there seems to be no harm in exploring cannabinoid therapies for skin conditions, including ones that I haven't had experience in treating. We have no evidence of harm or clinical concern with patients exploring these therapies. Use the same experimentation model we've discussed throughout the book: start your frequency and formulations low and slow, and advance your dosage over weeks, and possibly months, before you come to definitive conclusions.

If you have tried a product in the past and didn't get the results you were looking for, it's worth exploring entirely different formulations. Where THC is illegal to include in products, manufacturers have been adding CBD as the active cannabinoid in the topicals they produce. In states where THC is legal, product producers instead infuse THC as the active ingredient. The result is a thriving and varied market of topicals. You may find that for your condition, the THC-dominant products will be more effective, while for others, the CBD-rich varieties are preferable.

Treating Skin and Inflammation

Cannabinoids not only impact tissue function locally, they also affect cellular communication that travels between organ systems, such as the immune system, the nervous system, and the effects of mental health concerns on physical health. Some skin conditions seem to be rooted in the actions occurring in each of these three systems. It's no secret that mental stress and acne are linked. In the case of excessive inflammation, cannabis products show astounding success combating both the bacteria and the inflammation associated with acne and rosacea, as well as the effects of fungal overgrowth in athlete's foot, jock itch, and the rashes that often appear in armpits or under the breast. Cannabis has a protective role in all inflammatory skin conditions, ranging from allergic reactions like contact dermatitis, hives, and eczema to autoimmune conditions such as vitiligo and psoriasis.[3]

Cannabis can be used to treat autoimmune skin disorders by balancing the communication channels that keep inflammation in check. For example, psoriasis and eczema are two distinct inflammatory autoimmune disorders in which the immune system is fighting its own skin tissues. However, while either may show up in one area of the body or another, it's really a whole-body problem. That's why a treatment like cannabis, which affects the whole body when taken systemically, is going to be more effective, because you're addressing inflammation system-wide. You can certainly use topical cannabis as well, to address the local manifestation and local discomfort, and promote healing more quickly, while you are using it systemically to address the root cause of the malady.

If there is excessive activity in the skin, as with an overactive immune system, you might imagine that turning off immunity in the region would be curative. However, if your immunity were cut off entirely, bacteria, fungal, or viral invaders might escape this critical instrument of the body's defense, and would thrive and cause equal, if not greater, damage or illness. Cannabis offers the same balanced approach to inflammation that it does to receptor activation: at times activating immunity and at times calming it. Over the course of time, and under such conditions of balance, skin tissues slowly come to a new, healthy equilibrium, whereby the material that does not belong is gradually removed, and healthy tissues remain sustained and strong.

This mechanism is particularly important in cases of psoriasis. While we know the body is built to be a self-replacing system, when tissues are injured, the system of stem cells replaces them. However, the replacement cells occur before the underlying issue is healed and inflammation is still rampant. The cannabinoid system addresses both issues at the same time: calming inflammation and the autoimmune response that causes the psoriasis, while enhancing the activity of stem cells to produce more, new, and healthier tissues.

Blocking Bacteria, Fungi, and Viral Offenders

Your skin has barrier functions that prevent the outside world from getting inside, including toxins, allergens, and other invaders. For instance, dry skin is a leading cause of other skin diseases and symptoms. Cannabis lotions and creams can directly affect the fat production in sebaceous glands (either enhancing production or limiting it), thereby promoting healing from within the body, as well as amplifying the exterior barrier protection.[4]

As an antibacterial, antifungal, and antiviral treatment, cannabis can protect the skin and assist in healing wounds by directly eliminating the offenders that may try to penetrate this first line of defense.[5] It also strengthens the barrier function of the skin so that fewer microbes can get through.[6] At the cell wall itself, cannabinoids have been shown to impede cellular engagement with the offenders, preventing their invasion inside the cells. Lastly, there is evidence that shows that cannabinoids impact the cellular machinery, preventing unwanted microbes from replicating inside the cell.[7] It is through this same series of mechanisms that researchers have shown why cannabis may prevent and treat infectious diseases, such as COVID-19.[8]

For example, the rash that occurs when you come into contact with poison ivy shows how the skin's barrier function is broken by an irritating plant oil. The presence of this oil, urushiol, creates a local and regional inflammatory response, causing bumps, redness, itching, and occasionally pain. Cannabis topicals help to regulate the inflammatory response, physically coat the area to minimize the spread of urushiol, and stimulate rapid healing from the deep tissues in the skin by moisturizing and stimulating stem cells.

Cannabis as Sunscreen

The cannabis plant is rich in natural UV protection, which is how we know it can be used as a sunscreen. Picture a hailstorm, where some people have umbrellas and others don't. Cannabis acts like the umbrella, protecting the people underneath, whether it's taken topically or systemically.

Cannabis molecules applied directly to the skin are ideally shaped to enhance the skin's barrier function by deflecting damaging UV light. When cannabis is consumed systemically, its molecules are floating among blood cells, continuing its protection against incoming radiation. When the sun hits our skin and happens to penetrate that first line of defense, cannabis molecules neutralize the radiation and dissipate it.

This sun-protective feature is found in many terpene molecules across the plant kingdom. We should all aim to eat a diet dominated by fruits and vegetables. Until then, consider cannabis as an easily consumable option with similar sun-protection powers.

Cannabis Enhances the Skin's Motor, Sensory, and Transport Functions

The skin's motor function helps to regulate blood vessel dilation, which is a critical component of keeping the body at the right temperature and necessary for maintaining proper blood pressure. The movement of the tiny hairs that cover the body may trap heat or promote cooling, and the production of oil and sweat allows for another mechanism of temperature regulation. When these systems don't function properly, such as in anhidrosis or hyperhidrosis (too little or too much sweating), or when microbes cross through the skin and enter the bloodstream, the results can be deadly. Through its ability to moderate inflammation and support barrier function of both the skin and our immune system, topical and/or systemic cannabis options can facilitate optimal conditions for blood transport.

This motor function impacts the skin's ability to deliver nutrients and remove waste from one layer of the skin to another. Illnesses such as varicose veins or Raynaud's represent inconsistent blood flow and present as painful, swollen, discolored extremities. In both of these cases, topical cannabis therapies help correct imbalances of blood flow, stimulate healing of deep tissues, reduce pain, and strengthen regional immunity as they balance the inflammatory response.

Skin also affects sensory function. The nerve endings in the skin recognize touch, pressure, and temperature, as well as pain and itch. There are innumerable illnesses related to the skin's sensory function, including nerves that misfire or deliver the wrong signals. Skin burns or blistering illnesses can lead to nerve damage, as well as pain. In shingles, nerves beneath the skin are infected with the herpes virus and become painful, and the skin around them erupts in an uncomfortable regional rash. In diabetes, for example, excessive sugar causes damage to blood vessels and nerves, numbing skin sensation, causing the loss of hair from tense, inflamed tissues, and the restriction of healthy blood flow to support repair. Cannabis's unique ability to both heal skin and nerves (addressing nerve pain, neuropathy, as well as overall nerve functioning from the skin to the brain), and bring blood sugar levels under control, either topically or systemically, makes it unlike other nerve-related treatments.

Smoking Cannabis Is Not Ideal for Keeping Skin Youthful

If you're reading this chapter because your concern is aging skin and wrinkles, it's fair to say that smoking cannabis is not your best option. In fact, smoking is going to make wrinkles worse. The process of smoking actually ages skin: the temperature of smoke, the deprivation of oxygen, and the presence of toxic carbon monoxide all combine to dehydrate skin, rob it of its nutrients, and starve it from a healthy blood supply. Even vaporizing isn't ideal: the temperature from a vaporized product is lower than a flame but it does produce tar, which affects the quality of your teeth. When you smoke or vape, the tar, a sticky oil in microscopic spheres, gets aerosolized. When tar globules stick to your couch or your clothing, you will smell it. When they stick to your teeth, it finds its way into the tiny crevices in teeth, discoloring the surface, causing tooth decay, and damaging your gums.

Smoking cannabis can also cause dryness for the mucosal tissues in the mouth that are meant to stay moist with saliva. Salivation is one of the first-line protections against gum and tooth decay, and pure THC products directly affect mucosal membranes, leading to dried salivary glands, which causes cotton mouth; dry, red eyes; and increased appetite.

Your skin is not going to age prematurely with topicals or edibles that have a substantial CBD component. While some may say that they are not as effective as smoking, they are certainly effective.

Regimens for Skin Issues

The category of skin issues covers an incredibly wide range of symptoms and conditions. It is impossible that even a handful of suggested regimens could meet everyone's individual needs. However, what I can say is that for the vast majority of my patients with skin conditions, they see quick results. For my patients struggling with chronic acne, I have heard that topicals work within days. For others with excessive sweating or nerve pain, the results can be felt within minutes. Other conditions, such as wrinkles, scarring, vitiligo, or tumors, may take weeks or months for a change to be realized. Set your expectations depending on how deeply your skin tissues have been affected.

Then, answer the following questions to determine how to pick the right products:

1. Is your skin condition acute or chronic? Chronic conditions, including rashes that last more than a week, will benefit from longer-acting products, such as edibles or patches.

2. Are your symptoms persistent or intermittent (do they come and go)? Persistent symptoms may be better served with an edible; if they are intermittent, a topical might suffice. Topicals can be reapplied every few hours without worrying about hitting a maximum dose. You can cover topicals with a barrier that prevents evaporation or soiling your sheets or clothes. I often recommend wrapping the skin with Saran wrap or similar cling film to promote greater absorption after covering affected areas with topicals. Bandages applied to smaller areas, or gloves on hands, work as well.

3. Are your skin issues related to another health issue? For ideal results, address both the discomfort and the cause simultaneously. Many patients ultimately find success using both systemic and topical products.

Skin Product Recommendations

+ **Product recommendation #1—Topicals:** My patients seem uniformly pleased with the success of topicals compared to any other therapy to treat their skin concerns. Even when they are THC prominent, the formulations almost never have euphoric effects. In fact, their broader effects typically spread to no more than twelve inches from where they are applied. The commercial market seems to produce mainly weakly infused products; read labels to make sure you are getting a ratio of at least 100 mg of cannabis to every ounce of finished product. If you can't find what you need, you can always make your own (see chapter four). For example, coconut oil can be used as a base for hair products: many of my patients are applying it to the scalp to treat dandruff and stimulate the cells in the scalp to achieve hair growth. The mainstay of therapy for alopecia, the medical condition of hair loss, is injection of steroidal anti-inflammatories. If you have an anti-inflammatory like cannabis, which is stronger than steroids, it is reasonable to experiment and put it there and see what happens. In fact, a recent study has demonstrated that CB1 receptor antagonists do, indeed, induce hair growth in mice.[9]

+ **Product recommendation #2—Cannabis cooking oil/body oil applied directly:** This option offers a more concentrated dosage of cannabinoids compared to a diluted balm. Oils provide more relief that lasts longer. However, oils can be messy and expensive, and do not fully penetrate the skin, leaving the skin feeling sticky.

+ **Product recommendation #3—Skin patches:** Patches offer a discrete, long-lasting diffusion of cannabinoids through the skin. They are not euphoric and require less frequent reapplication; one patch can last as long as twelve hours. Place the patch near the affected area: if you are dealing with acne, for example, place the patch on the back of your neck or on your chest.

Cannabis and Medications

If you feel that your traditional skin treatments aren't working, the unique nature of cannabis products makes them an exceptional therapy and worth trying. Their effects will also amplify traditional skin medicines. For example, added to an athlete's foot medication, cannabis topicals may add a greater antifungal effect than each medication would provide individually. Do not stop taking prescription medications without fully consulting your prescribing healthcare provider. You should feel comfortable with cannabis and how it might make you feel before you entertain reducing other medicines or getting off them.

CHAPTER 14

Sexual Function and Sexual Health

B arbara came to see me with what she thought was an unusual request. As a sixty-eight-year-old woman who was deeply in love with her husband, she shared that her sexual experiences had been unfulfilling her whole life. She had long found sex to be extremely painful, and she had terrible anxiety every time her spouse, Jack, suggested it.

I told Barbara that her issue is, unfortunately, not all that unusual. In fact, I have met dozens of women like her over the years. I reminded her that sexuality isn't just about body parts and hormones, although these building blocks are surely one aspect of it, and that cannabis could impact her physical and mental discomforts. I assured Barbara that she would be able to address her concerns discreetly, as we talked about the impressive results other women have reported with cannabis-based therapies. Barbara pursued a topical lubricant that would both relax the tense musculature in her genitalia and amplify the natural lubrication that many women lose after menopause. I also suggested that she take a single THC-dominant edible candy about forty-five minutes prior to having sex, which would help her feel less uneasy and perhaps more playful.

When she called me a week later to check in, she informed me that she found the lubricant that I had suggested at a local dispensary and bought out the entire inventory. For the first time, she was able to enjoy sex to the fullest. Then Barbara told me that she asked the distributor to order more so that she could share the good news and the opportunity with her girlfriends. The edible did help some, but the topical is what really moved her from pain to pleasure.

For many men and women, good sex is elusive, regardless of their choice in partner, or comfort with sexual acts or expression. Chronic conditions like heart disease, diabetes, obesity, and arthritis can constrain sexual performance. Older women may find sex uncomfortable or anxiety-producing after menopause. Other women have experienced years of sexual difficulty, including suffering from conditions like vaginismus or vulvodynia, both of which are diagnoses related to extreme sensitivity to touch and penetration at and into the vagina. Men often face challenges with physical stamina, sustaining erections, ejaculation disorders, and inhibited sexual desire.

At some point, nearly everyone experiences uneasiness or discomfort around sex. The experience may spark apprehension or panic related to the vulnerability that sex presents. Or the process may include the absence of pleasure or the presence of pain. Many people are distracted during sex by their own concerns of low self-esteem, which can affect their performance. I've also heard many individuals express frustration that sex would be more appealing if their partner was more present and attentive to their needs.

Fortunately, guided cannabis therapies have shown to enhance sexual function, improve sexual health, and provide the space to build deeper, loving relationships. This is true for both men and women.

As we learned in chapter four, each of us interacts with cannabis products differently, and within our own set and setting. When people come together during sex, another layer of complexity is added to the mix. Keep in mind that the product that enhances your sexual experience may not affect your partner in the same way, or at all. Finding what products work best for each of you, both separately and when you are together, can only enhance the overall experience.

A Note About Gender Identification

This book was written in a time of cultural change, when the definitions of male, female, and fluid gender identities are evolving to be inclusive. The discussions in this chapter will refer to "male" and "female," "men," and "women," in an effort to explain the interactions between cannabis, the human body, and hormones, so that you can see how enhancing your endocannabinoid system impacts fertility and the sexual response cycles. From this vantage point, you will be able to relate the information to your particular needs, sexual identity, and unique preferences.

Cannabis Improves Sexual Response

The sexual response is, in many ways, the exact intersection where cannabis therapies do best: it is a meeting place of the mind and the body. There are aspects of sexual relationships that are physical, components that are emotional, and elements that manifest somewhere between strict biology and psychology, relating to the social dynamics between two consenting adults.

You have already learned that cannabis can decrease anxiety, increase forgetfulness, and increase sensory perception. Cannabinoids increase libido by stabilizing mood and creating an environment of warmth, positivity, and cognitive centeredness, which is not only a pause from distractions, but also a forgetfulness of negative thoughts that you may have about sex or about the circumstances. It also provides an ability to be more aware and present during sexual activity. Couples who use cannabis together can share an experience of novelty and sensory enhancement, which often adds to their sexual excitement. And cannabinoids can either stimulate or blunt the release of numerous hormones that play a role in mediating sexual interest, sexual preparedness, and behaviors. For example, cannabinoids increase the firing rate of oxytocin, the "feel good" brain chemical released during sexual stimulation and orgasm. They also contribute directly to deepening feelings of love and bonding.[1] With more oxytocin available, sex becomes more relational and less transactional: We get cuddlier and less goal-oriented. That change in perspective alone can make for better sexual relations.

These facets, taken together, can increase one's experience of joy. With an open attitude, you may find that cannabis allows you to tap into sexual desires that have always been available to you, although not necessarily accessible, leading to an increased motivation to seek out sexual encounters and deepen existing relationships.[2,3] It's not surprising to me that people who consume cannabis regularly have more sex, and they feel proud and confident in their sexuality. These effects are consistent across age groups, which means that good sex is available to you throughout your lifetime. In my practice, I see hundreds of men and women up into their eighties who are enjoying regular, fulfilling sexual encounters.

Enhancing the Physical Aspects of Sex

On the physical side, the actions of the endocannabinoid system affect sex in many distinct ways. First, the anti-inflammatory action helps to increase blood flow to the skin, nerves, and muscles at erogenous areas, presenting the opportunity to experience amplified sensitivity to touch during consensual sexual encounters. The interaction of cannabinoids with nerves, some of which increase signal strength while others slow down communication, focuses and increases sensory perception, which can add an element of novelty and excitement to sexual contact.

The smooth muscle relaxation action of cannabis makes sex more comfortable for everyone. In one study on women, those who used cannabis before sex noted a decrease in pain and improved orgasms.[4] The exertional aspects of sex naturally build muscle tension, fatigue, and sometimes spasm. Just as patients report improved tolerance and shortened recovery times during general fitness exercises when cannabis is on board, the same effects apply to the muscles that are taxed during intercourse.

Cannabis is known to increase heart rate and blood flow.[5] With a cannabinoid product on board, blood flow is directed to the genitals, which can improve erections in men and female sexual arousal. This increased genital blood flow enhances sensitivity at the nerve endings in the penis and vagina during physical stimulation. Enhanced circulation may also amplify the immersive nature of sexual experience at both the body level and in the mind, as increased heart rate is often associated with deeper emotional connections.[6]

Sex hormones, including estrogen and testosterone, help define physical and sexual characteristics. Men and women have variable amounts of both hormones. Cannabis is thought to increase the availability of the sex hormone testosterone,[7] which we know makes both men and women more libidinous. A second consequence of enhanced testosterone availability is an increase in the hormone adrenaline, which is another vital component in the physiology of the sexual response. The presence of adrenaline during sex can increase your level of excitement and arousal, which adds to relationship bonding.[8]

Your current physical health, including the medications that you are taking, may also affect your sexual response and performance. For example, many illnesses, including depression, anxiety, heart disease, diabetes, or conditions like arthritis, chronic pain, and menstrual pain—and the medications used to treat them—can affect one's ability to be intimate. While you should not stop taking your medication for potential sexual benefit alone, adding cannabis to your existing regimen may help ease your overall physical discomfort and improve sexual function at the same time. By treating both your sexual concerns and other illnesses with cannabis, you may be able to go back to an activity—sex—that brings you joy and stress relief, potentially building a cycle of benefits.

The sheer presence of a cannabis product, whether euphoric, gently calming, or simply offering peace of mind through simple reduction in physical discomfort, can affect sex powerfully. In small amounts, cannabis products may enable someone to be more social, feel more content, generally be more comfortable with themselves and their circumstances, and more easily open themselves up to others sexually. For many of my patients, cannabis offers a period of mental stillness and welcome vacation from the day's usual thought patterns, and it becomes a way to temporarily escape the pesky details and nagging thoughts of a stressful daily life. As people have discovered that cannabis helps them separate work life from home life, the opportunity for intimacy and availability at home also grows. Once someone is free of the demands of modern life, the natural instincts to seek pleasure and tension release often prevail. This is because the presence of cannabis is not merely supporting the body's natural proclivity to sexual activity, by consistently enhancing levels of testosterone or estrogen flowing through the veins, but the presence of cannabis also brings with it all of the systematic effects that can contribute positively to sexuality: a sense of calm and contentment, comfort in the body, relaxation in the mind, and emotional stability, all with acceptable, if not desirable, side effects.

There Are Good Reasons to Have More Sex

There are a host of long-term benefits of having frequent sexual relations: it's good for resetting the brain by enhancing cognitive function, improving sleep, and reducing mental stress. We also know that it's good for heart health and your immune system.[9] For men, frequent sex decreases the risk of prostate cancer.[10] For women, one study showed that weekly sexual encounters can increase telomere length, a biological feature linked to longevity.[11]

Antidepressants and Sexual Function

Sex hormones are governed by a cascade system that starts in the brain. In a series of sequential steps that feed one on the other, this cascade ultimately leads to the production of local hormones in the ovaries or testes. But when you medically adjust the chemistry at the top of the cascade, it will change the hormone production of the entire system. That's why some people who are taking antidepressants may feel less depressed, but with fewer hormones available, they may also develop symptoms of sex hormone imbalance, such as weight gain or acne, or find that they are less interested in having sex and/or have difficulty achieving an orgasm.

For many, cannabinoids provide a different, more appealing alternative to antidepressants, alleviating the heaviness of depression without affecting the hormone cascade manifestations that they don't want. If you remain on the antidepressants, cannabis can help reverse the hormonal and sexual side effects. If you can get off antidepressants using cannabis as a bridge, your normal level of sexual interest will return. And if you opt to replace antidepressants with a regular cannabis regimen, your sexual interest may be greater, and more enjoyable, than it was before.

Cannabis and Fertility

One aspect of sexual health to consider before using cannabis is the impact that it may have on fertility. Strong research confirms that the endocannabinoid system affects both men and women at every stage of fertility: the generation and growth of a female's reproductive follicles, a male's sperm, the process of fertilization, the transportation of ovum, and the processes of implantation and embryo development. The fact of the endocannabinoid system's involvement is not a subject of debate, but how the elements of reproduction are impacted—whether for better or worse, what opportunities there may be to assist with fertility challenges, and what opportunities there may be to identify new means of birth control—is an area of exciting ongoing research. One aspect of investigation is the quality of semen when cannabis is involved. Some studies show that sperm swim slower and less effectively, and their numbers are reduced.[12] The same is true for the fimbriae that line the fallopian tube; these are the microscopic, fingerlike projections of tissue that line the fallopian tube, which help to move an egg closer to the uterus. When certain forms of cannabis are on board, the fimbriae appear to be less efficient, and there is a greater risk of failed or ectopic pregnancy.[13]

While these studies seem to show that cannabis inhibits fertility, I see them in a slightly different light. In the setting of a culture that has, for generations, demonized the use of cannabis, science has identified and repeatedly publicized an association between reduced fertility and cannabis use. Rather than interpreting the relationship as an association, and with appropriate uncertainty—perhaps couples were consuming cannabis to cope with their reproductive challenges, or experimenting with cannabis as a treatment for fertility—a bias promoting the perceived harms of cannabis has systematically linked cannabis and infertility.

Instead, I would argue that the overall effect changes the outcome only in a very low percentage. It's possible that people who are consuming cannabis are more libidinous, and they're having more sex, and typically report more enjoyable experiences. This increased rate of sexual interaction may counterbalance the decreased function. So even if there is a small detriment to sperm motility or to fallopian tube motility, the overall effect is that there is actually increased fertility. This perspective is supported by public health and epidemiological data that I've researched, which consistently show that regions of the world with high rates of cannabis use do not report reduced rates of fertility.

This example spotlights an important vulnerability present in modern science: there is often a hazardous disconnect between small-scale investigations and outcomes-based data that takes a larger, more comprehensive perspective. This is an immense challenge that has tarnished the public's perception of medicinal cannabis for generations: the microscopic views are often unflattering, but the large-scale prohibition of cannabis has made macroscopic studies challenging to perform. As consumers, we're left with a skewed understanding, which often excludes a more holistic point of view.

Increasing Both Joy and Pleasure

Cannabis is keenly disinhibiting, often more than alcohol. Many of my patients report a renewed—and sometimes completely new—desire to experience pleasure while consuming cannabis. With cannabis on board, you may find that you are interested in exploring your own body's sensitivity.

Self-pleasure is available to everyone: cannabis is simply providing a freeing opportunity to explore your body in a safe environment. Particularly when cannabis is included in the experience, solo sex is an opportunity to learn and explore your likes and discover heightened sensations or altered perspectives. The opportunity to alter your perspective, in a setting of your own control, adds unequaled value to building a healthy relationship with others.

Addressing the Symptoms of Menopause

During menopause, women have enormous hormonal instability, which leads to hot flashes, increased anxiety, poor sleep, and a general lack of comfort, including diminishing vaginal lubrication during sex. While we have already reviewed throughout the book cannabis's positive influences on reducing anxiety, improving sleep, and resolving pain, it can also alleviate the symptoms that are primarily related to menopause. While there is no direct data that suggests that cannabinoids specifically reduce hot flashes, many of my menopausal patients have shared with me that using cannabinoids has brought them meaningful, although often temporary, relief. I often recommend lotions for women to use on the chest and abdomen to turn down the volume of hot flashes. Systemic options that are transmitted via the bloodstream, such as edibles and tinctures, can reach both local regions and have meaningful impact on soothing anxiety; increasing the ability to sleep; improving the consistency of deep, restful sleep; and providing support for genital discomfort.

A Cautionary Warning for Male Sexual Health

The goal of cannabis therapies is to enhance normal physiology and sex hormone production and availability. For some men with hormonal deficiencies or other illnesses, enhancement can return their sexual function to a normal state. For men who already have healthy sexual function, a temporary enhancement can be pleasurable, but prolonged exposure to cannabinoids may have negative repercussions. At low doses, cannabis helps libido and erectile function, but at high doses with consistent use, it may have the opposite effect, albeit on a temporary basis.[14] Too much cannabis at one time can also lead to paranoia and anxiety, which, as you might expect, would also inhibit male orgasm and pleasure.

Be aware of the interactions between your sexual function and cannabis use, and make adjustments when you experience a physical or mental reaction that is not aligned with your wishes. With all the positive impacts that cannabis can have, it's important to remember that over long periods of time, too much of a good thing is really too much.

MEET SAM

Getting to the right dosage is critically important. For instance, my patient Sam is a successful, mature man in his midfifties who is very busy and doesn't have a lot of time for seeking sexual encounters. However, when he does, he told me that he doesn't feel as skillful as he did when he was younger. He knows that he doesn't have the physique that he used to, and that in his every-day life he's overworked and stressed out. He came to see me when a recent sexual encounter ended with erectile dysfunction. I explained to Sam that cannabis could help him reduce his anxiety and increase erectile function at the same time. He was happy to know that he had options that were less spon-taneous and awkward compared to the "Blue Pill," and I told him to report back in a few weeks to let me know how things were going.

A month later, Sam came back with a tale of mixed results. At first, his sexual relations were noticeably more comfortable and fulfilling. He was motivated to socialize and have sex more often, because he was feeling more relaxed in general, and he felt a much more satisfying separation of his work from his social life. However, after two weeks of daily, high-dosage use, it seemed like the magic had faded. The novelty of cannabis wasn't addressing his erectile dysfunction. Perhaps unrelated stressors may have been revived, or perhaps Sam had developed a tolerance to the low dose of full-spectrum, 2:1 CBD:THC product that he was taking by flower vaporizer. After reviewing the many possible contributing factors, we devised a plan together for him to increase his cannabis dosage incrementally, and to add some dedicated time to his daily routine for strength-training exercises that might help him to lose weight, to further separate work from home time, and also boost natural testosterone levels. To Sam's surprise and frustration, the product I recom-mended was sold out. I taught Sam to use his vaporizer device to precisely control temperature, and he was able to capture a more desirable mixture of CBD in the flower he already had, until the product I recommended was back in stock. We also purchased a supply of pure CBD flower along with a supply of THC flower so that he could sustain his preferred ratio regardless of dispensary stocking issues.

Regimens for Better Sex

In the absence of feelings of joy, pleasure, and contentment, my patients often lean on cannabis to provide some of these missing finishes. In such a situation, one might imagine that products of almost any type could remedy the deficiency. Yet, in my experience, treating individuals with endocannabinoid deficiency requires as much trial and error as any other type of cannabis therapy. While some patients find localized application of topicals pleasure enhancing, others benefit from the emotional effects of systemic cannabis more than regional uses. As with most elements within cannabis medicine, different forms of cannabis can address different aspects of emotional or relational or physical contact, and the best match depends as much on the nuances of the patient's day-to-day environment as it does on their overall health.

+ **Onset timing:** When it comes to sex, fast-acting products work quickly: you can expect to use them right away, as part of a sexual encounter. These products are a good match for enhancing sexual function if these issues are acute or intermittent. Products meant to have rapid effects bring an instant relief of expectation and gratification that has manifold benefit. For chronic sexual dysfunction and those situations where there is a known medical diagnosis being addressed through traditional channels, consistent dosing, in the low to moderate range, seems to be more effective over time than quick actors.

+ **Short-acting versus longer-lasting:** Men who struggle with performance anxiety, or other emotional causes of reduced interest in sexuality, tend to benefit from systemic delivery choices such as edibles, tinctures, and suppositories. For men and women who suffer from either erectile dysfunction, anorgasmia, or reduced genital sensation, topicals can be quite effective. For women, topicals applied to genitalia (administered by bath bomb, regional balms, or lubricants) appear to be more effective than for men. This is perhaps because of the advantage that women have in the increased availability of mucosal tissue, which allows for larger dosages to cross into the body.

+ **Euphoric/non-euphoric:** As much as we would like it to be true, there is no specific strain or product that is guaranteed to deliver better sex. The answer is whatever works best for you.

+ **Terpenes:** Some terpene components found in cannabis seem to enhance libido through a very specific increase in sexual desire. These include limonene, linalool, caryophyllene, humulene, and terpinolene. If you cannot find products that include these terpenes, consider preparing a very dilute solution of safety-tested terpene product that can be purchased online to an existing lubricant (one drop terpene to five drops coconut oil).

+ **Product recommendation—personal lubricants:** Topical cannabinoids have been specifically formulated as sexual lubricants. The added value these products offer is the ability to relax the genital musculature with an effective systemic relaxation, a combination that more easily yields enhanced sexual gratification beyond lubrication. The same lubricants can be used for men and women, although each absorbs topicals differently. Some older women find topicals irritating, particularly those that are THC-dominant. Anything that is not balanced for the vagina specifically is going to sting, and that's a feature of the base lotion product and not a feature of cannabis. There are an increasing number of CBD products that are marketed specifically to men or women. As with all products purchased online, look for laboratory-tested products from companies that value medical and/or scientific leadership. If you're going to make a lubricant, use a lubricating product that you have had experience using for sexual activity before, and add cannabis oil to it to enhance the effectiveness. See chapter four for lubricant recipes.

MEET BRYAN

Bryan was infected with hepatitis B through sexual contact in 2014. His primary care provider brought it to his attention during a routine physical, and he was quickly referred to a gastroenterologist. By that time, his infection was considered to be chronic and was affecting his liver function. His bloodwork showed that he had already developed some cirrhosis.

Bryan qualified to enter a drug study to help find a cure for hep B. It lasted for a year, during which time he received twelve injections over a six-month span, as well as the medication Tenofovir D. The side effects of pain and nausea were extremely difficult to tolerate. Bryan instinctively knew that there must be a way to deal with his side effects, which is what brought him to my office.

Bryan had already explored low-dose edibles, available mixtures of CBD and THC, and was smoking flower. Each of these individual options was not providing enough coverage for his side effects. Instead, we developed a plan to start microdosing an alcohol-extracted Full Extract Cannabis Oil (FECO) sold as Rick Simpson Oil (RSO). I explained that this product had particularly strong euphoric effects, and the only way it could be tolerated during the day is through a series of small dosages. Yet, this protocol means that each dose is both strong and short-lasting. To create a more sustained effectiveness, I typically prescribe it alongside other cannabis products. What's more, using a blend of diverse products, each with their own cannabinoid ingredients, works to create effects that don't appear when each product is consumed individually. This phenomenon is known as the *entourage effect,* or what I call an *emergence effect.* Bryan could then dose the RSO at the same time as taking other tinctures, edibles, and flower to vape during the day, to get the best results. At night, he could forgo the microdosing entirely and choose a longer-lasting product.

Once we found a RSO dose that suited his tolerance to THC, he was able to comfortably manage the side effects of his treatment. What's more, his liver function test numbers returned to safe levels relatively quickly. We never expected that cannabis could treat his liver function, as these effects had not been reported in the medical literature. We were pleasantly surprised to see that within a month of starting a cannabis regimen, Bryan had completely reversed his cirrhosis and restored his liver function. In fact, he was responding better than the study's researchers could explain; they admitted this rapid decline in inflammation within the liver was not their doing. His kidneys, which had also shown signs of inflammation, returned to normal as well.

Even with this positive outcome, it is still in Bryan's best interest to remain on some form of antiviral therapy to keep his hep B under control. However, he can continue to take the medication with cannabis to combat the debilitating side effects of treatment. Nine years later, his bloodwork remains perfect and he has achieved an undetectable viral load.

Not only has cannabis helped his health, it has led Bryan on a healing journey that has changed his life. Because of his positive experience with cannabis, he has become open to other nontraditional therapies and embraces an overall healing lifestyle. His experience has taught me that being open to accept the unexpected can lead to better medical outcomes than we ever thought were possible.

CHAPTER 15

Treating Cancer and the Symptoms of Traditional Cancer Therapies

T he conversation surrounding cancer and cannabis is complex. It's very different from many of the other disease processes we've reviewed because cannabis can alleviate the symptoms associated with the traditional treatments of the disease, and may, in fact, be able to act independently to address the disease processes themselves. However, there's one important caveat to state up front: there is little reliable scientific research that shows, in people, that cannabis is an effective treatment for cancer. The science that does exist is not well documented or supported and has not passed yet another critical step for it to be trustworthy: reproducibility. Most of the impressive research has been conducted on the microscopic level, in petri dishes, looking at how cancer cells respond to the presence of different cannabinoids.

Yet, over the years, I have seen firsthand clinical data that makes me optimistic. I have counseled hundreds of patients who would appear to have impossibly good luck, if it weren't for their use of cannabis. These patients have dealt with the full range of cancers at various stages: single organ issues, multiple organ growths, small skin cancers, cancers that are riddled throughout the body, and some diagnoses that, to a traditional modern medical view, are believed to be incurable. So many of them are doing great, meaning that they are completely cancer-free, as long as they stay the course and remain on cannabis treatments.

The types of people who seek cannabis treatments are invariably approaching cannabis therapies from different phases of their disease. Almost universally, they are continuing with their traditional cancer treatments—which I encourage unequivocally—but are looking for something to augment their primary therapy. Many of my patients are older adults or people who have received a terminal diagnosis, and they are generally looking for *palliation*, or symptom management related to treatments like chemotherapy or radiation. Sometimes they want to increase their appetite, because they have no interest in eating anymore. Some of them have pain or intolerable nauseousness. Many are so uncomfortable, from many possible causes, that they need help getting to sleep and taking a break from persistent depression or anxiety.

A second group of patients are in the fighting phase: they want to live and will do whatever it takes to stay alive, even when they know that they are approaching the end of the road. Many in this group have heard about "miraculous" cannabis treatments that worked when all other options have failed, or they watched the 2018 feature film *Weed the People*, which highlighted a handful of families with children who had cancer, portraying surprising successes in the face of what seemed like inescapable misfortune.

The third group are people who have been recently diagnosed. They may be younger and optimistic, and often are at the earliest stages of the disease and facing an overwhelming array of treatment choices. They are looking to treat the disease and prevent the worst of the symptoms related to treatment. A large portion of this group seems to think skeptically about the traditional medical system and prefers a more "natural" treatment.

No matter where you or a loved one is on the cancer journey, there is a role for cannabis that merits serious consideration. In this chapter, I will help you to understand the anecdotal evidence that supports cannabis, especially in the late stages of cancer. To my mind, you have nothing to lose with this experiment—and everything to gain.

Cannabis Can Help You Make Good
Decisions About Your Diagnosis

We are fortunate to live in a time when adults are doing better with cancer diagnoses. There are very few cancers that attack organs that are beyond treatment. Outside of pancreatic and brain cancers, almost all forms of cancer occur in places where people can continue to live well without a particular organ (as in breast or ovarian cancer) or can manage their health pharmacologically. Yet there is still tremendous anxiety associated with any diagnosis, which is the first place where cannabis can help.

Not only does cannabis distract you from rumination and worry; it helps you look at your life through a different lens. When we are faced with a traumatic diagnosis like cancer, it's very difficult to think clearly. Some people might think that having cannabis on board can lead to bad decision-making, but I think it actually can do the opposite: it can help you tune out distractions, including your emotional turmoil, so that you can understand the situation with clarity and focus.

For instance, it can be hard to assess the major priorities of life immediately after hearing a diagnosis, and you may want to think about "big picture" issues: *What does my family want for the long term? What are the realistic cost limitations that we have? What do I still want to do in my life?* Cannabis can help you shift out of the scenery of everyday life and open up a space where you can really think about a serious change in those variables. Cannabis can also help you turn down the volume of extreme emotions, so that real decision-making is more approachable. Turning down the dial can help you detach from the emotional angst that may be in the ether of input from well-intentioned family and friends. When the outside world is quieter, and when your focus is extreme, it's an easier space to be thoughtful and present.

How Cannabis May Treat Cancers

Any type of cancer represents a physical cluster of cells. If cannabis is doing good work to kill a cancer or to stop it from moving or replicating, it has to do it at the cellular level. One of cannabis's overarching actions is the reversal of cellular disruption. Cell death is a normal, healthy, expected part of a cell's life cycle: they are designed with an operating mechanism to self-destruct whenever they experience dysfunction, damage, infection, or some other catastrophic problem. This automatic cell self-destruction is known as *apoptosis*. If cellular functioning is damaged and leads to excessive growth and/or escaping apoptosis, a fast-growing, cancerous "zombie" cell is formed. As the cancer expands, it continues to avoid destruction, living long past when it should have been destroyed.

Cannabis can change the signaling, activating cell death by opening channels of communication where the cells can once again remember that they are supposed to self-destruct. By doing so, cancer growth is stopped.[1] In laboratory study, it appears that when cannabinoids are present, only the cancer cells activate self-elimination signaling, and surrounding healthy cells are totally unaffected.[2] That is a very different outcome compared to common chemotherapies, which tend to strike against all fast-growing cells, regardless of those cells' origin or damage. This is why many people shed their hair and eyebrows during chemotherapy: hair is comprised of fast-growing cells, which can be inadvertently attacked and killed off.

Cannabis also inhibits the number of new cancer cells by many different known mechanisms. When cancer cells are blossoming, or growing the same way our normal cells do, they are directed by communication signals to continue growing, to separate, divide, and produce new cells, in a process called *proliferation*. Cannabis offers the opportunity for interruption of typical cancer cell proliferation signals, at a genetic level.[3] The cannabis is not killing the cancer cell; it's impacting the process of normal cell life. Cannabis can also interrupt other stages of the proliferation process. At many stages of the life of a cancerous cell, it becomes less viable when cannabis is on board.[4]

Cancer is bad where it first develops, but it can be worse when it moves into other places within the body. Cellular invasion requires both the multiplication of cancer cells as well as the breakdown of the scaffolding that keeps cellular contents contained. This is accomplished, in part, by matrix metalloproteinases (MMPs), enzymes that live outside of cells that function like scissors cutting through a mesh bag of fruit, allowing cancer cells to enter. Some antibiotics use this mechanism to prevent infections from spreading; cannabinoids can also block MMPs from working properly at the cellular level for cancer.[5] Through this mechanism, cannabis can prevent the building blocks from moving cancer from one tissue to another.

Cancer growth can occur when there is an opening in the internal, cellular infrastructure, which allows cells to proliferate independent of their normal reproductive schedule. Laboratory research has shown that cannabis has the ability to stop cells from differentiation and prevent normal proliferation of cancer cells.[6]

When healthy cells are taken over by cancer, it is hardly business as usual within the cell. The invaded cells lose the process to self-clean. Cannabis is both helpful and harmful, as all immune cells bind cannabinoids. In some cases, those immune cells, some of which are there to kill cancer, will do their job. However, one of the critical roles of the immune system is to sound the alarm when things go wrong. When cannabis is present, this type of immunity is quieted, dampening both the local and system-wide alarms.[7]

Focus on Prostate Cancer

Prostate cancer provides a clear case study to show how cannabis can help address the symptoms of the disease, and possibly the disease itself. One of the most common symptoms of prostate cancer is nocturnal enuresis (bed-wetting). The sensation that leads to bladder emptying is a nerve and muscle problem. Cannabis can both quiet overactive nerves and restore muscle function. The overall effect for some men is better bladder control. Another symptom of prostate cancer is a persistent sensation of pressure, as the enlarged, cancer-filled tissue presses into nearby tissues. In these circumstances, cannabis can help soothe the relevant nerves or activated muscle tissues, so that feelings of pressure are relieved. Cannabis can also quell the anxiety associated with both bed-wetting and discomfort.

In terms of treating the disease, researchers are focusing on CBD and its anti-cancer activity. Prostate cancer cells have increased expression of cannabinoid receptors, which when stimulated, result in reduced viability of the cells, increased cell death, and a reduction in other hormones, which reduces the chance for the cancer to thrive.[8]

Regimens for Cancer Symptom Treatment

If you are considering cannabis therapies, there is an important choice to make: use cannabis to treat your symptoms, or attempt to treat the disease. The decision is ultimately driven by how aggressive you want to be. When my patients choose to consume high doses of cannabis, they often report experiencing meaningful impact at combating cancers. When patients choose lower doses, their experience may be more comfortable, but they will not obtain as much cancer-killing action. Many of my patients end up switching to higher doses in the hopes of maximizing their success.

It is not always the case, but many physical cancer symptoms are a result of the treatment. The following are the most common symptoms across all cancers that cannabis can address:[9]

+ **Fatigue and poor sleep:** With or without cancer, people who are worried, depressed, or in pain have trouble sleeping. Cancer treatments can cause all three of these underlying issues. As you learned in chapter seven, cannabis can act as a powerful agent to help you get to sleep and stay asleep. Better sleep will help offset daily lethargy, and cannabis can also help increase energy levels.

+ **Constipation, diarrhea, nausea, and loss of appetite:** Many cancer treatments cause nauseousness and stomach upset. In almost all cases I have seen, when someone is using cannabis along with a traditional anti-neoplastic chemotherapy, cannabis can treat GI issue side effects more effectively than any other pharmaceutical, and choices higher in THC can increase appetite. See chapter twelve for more information on specific treatment options, and choose products that you can tolerate and will stay in your system if you are frequently vomiting, like patches or suppositories. I've had patients who are in the ICU, and their caretakers were administering cannabis suppositories because they couldn't eat.

+ **Pain:** Cancer treatments can cause generalized and localized pain. Sometimes, the method of treatment is injections, which are painful at the injection site. Both chemotherapy and radiation kill the fast-growing tissues, including cells in the bones and skin, and when these cells/tissues die it is very painful. Recovery between treatments can also be painful, as your body has been traumatized. Cannabinoids bind to and activate mu opiate receptors, and they produce results that are in the same family as morphine, albeit dramatically less potent. Nonetheless, the pain relief is significant. See chapter eleven for more information on specific treatment options. For instance, topicals can be used to both prevent and heal the damage from radiation.

+ **Depression:** Living with cancer can be terrifying, often throwing the sufferer and their family into despair. It's frightening to imagine what's happening inside that is beyond your control, especially when you are living with a diagnosis. Consuming cannabis helps lift long-lasting depression, as well as provides on-demand relief that is simple, safe, and deeply comforting for addressing shorter-term surges in depression and anxiety.

Regimens for Cancer Treatment

Cannabis treatments for cancer are robust. Some traditional cancer medicines work by triggering downstream reactions where a small amount of medication creates a big result. Other medicines build a tone of persistent effect while the medicine is present. Cannabis appears to work by influencing the right tone. To do so, it is believed that a large volume of cannabis is needed to achieve this tonal change and make a lasting difference: if there are ten thousand pieces of cancer, it appears that you may need at least ten thousand pieces of cannabis to interact with localized cancer cells. This action is profoundly different from chemotherapy, which acts systemically to attack all fast-growing cells in the body. In some ways, the cannabis strategy is similar to how radiation therapy operates: a beam of electromagnetic radiation destroys the cancer cells with which it comes in direct contact. During a course of radiation, there are bound to be casualties of healthy cells inadvertently killed. Cannabis does not harm those bystanders the way that radiation does. While taken systemically, the killing action of cannabinoids is limited only to cancer cells.

The amount of cannabis you have to take in order to achieve a level of treatment is significantly more than what you need to get a good night's sleep or to address pain, and it may be physically and mentally unsettling at first, especially if someone is new to cannabis. With so much cannabis on board, you may not be able to function at the level that you're used to. You may experience a change in cognition that can noticeably impact your career and home life. Cannabis allows for cross-communication between different systems of the brain, which can lead to distraction for someone who is susceptible to distraction. It can also be hyper-focusing, leading to an inability to get "off task" or stop ruminating thoughts. However, once you develop a tolerance, these unpleasant feelings will go away, and you will eventually find that further increases in dosing are less likely to come with discomfort. Sarah, one of my breast cancer survivors, once told me, "I'm taking high doses on a daily basis, and I don't feel high anymore. My cancer seems to have stopped growing, and I can manage my daily life again. I'm feeling hopeful because this has been a different journey than I first expected."

The ultimate goal of cannabis cancer treatment is to achieve tolerance as the cancer goes away. If the cancer continues to grow and/or spread, you will have to continue to up the ante: try different cannabis strains or products, and try more of them. The approach to treatment is to consume a huge amount of a broad-spectrum flower—featuring both THC and CBD as well as many other cannabinoids—as quickly as you can tolerate. If one strain or product doesn't work, bring in another without discarding the first. The more variety you can handle at the same time, the better. Typically, my patients find that if they begin with a tolerable small dose and increase dosage incrementally and steadily, it is possible to achieve very high doses in a few weeks' time.

It's very difficult to ingest large volumes consistently merely by inhaling, and because combustion is destructive to the plant, smoking or vaping are recommendations of last resort. Most people end up consuming cannabinoid-rich oils in the form of cannabis-dense edibles or tinctures because they offer the highest concentration of cannabinoids in the smallest package. Commercially prepared edibles are often decarboxylated so that they are more stable to sell. For treating most illnesses, that's fine, but for cancer, the action of the pre-decarboxylated forms may be equal, if not more effective, to combat cancer. My advice is to make sure you get some of each to maximize your chances of success. Using flower from a dispensary, and making edibles from them, is recommended. You can put the dried flower directly into a blender with ingredients for your favorite smoothie to create a pre-decarboxylated edible. And you can create a cannabis oil or butter and cook with it to get the benefits of the decarboxylated forms. If you can purchase concentrate, you can put it in peanut butter. If you prefer swallowing pills, you can make your own pills by filling capsules with full-spectrum cannabis oil. Regardless of your choice, start with a tolerable dose and advance incrementally every time you take it. The good news is that, at higher doses, you will naturally be treating your symptoms as you go. Make sure to let your healthcare provider know that you are using high doses of THC so that they can accurately monitor your health.

Some people with cancer come to cannabis as their "Hail Mary" treatment option, when all other options seem futile. This approach usually leaves little buffer time to build up a comfortable tolerance. With a rushed effort to increase dosages too quickly, the process will be unpleasant and you may want to quit quickly. If cannabis is part of an early treatment discussion, the likelihood of success is stronger, because you will have a longer runway to better tolerate the treatment. Patients who are at early stages of cancer are likely to require smaller volumes of cannabis, and people who have larger tumors or who begin at later-stage cancers typically need more.

It appears that once you have found cancer-fighting success using cannabis, with or without traditional treatment plans, you can lower your level of consumption to create a maintenance dosage if you achieve remission. You will taper down the same way that you ramped up your dose: cut your dosage slightly every few days. While we don't know what an ideal maintenance dose is, my patients report that they can maintain a dosage level that is not too expensive, and is effective, at around 25 percent of their maximum dose.

However, if the cannabis treatment is fully withdrawn, cancer seems to return. We do not presently know why this occurs, but it has been confirmed by numerous doctors in my field. This means that when people use cannabis to fight cancer, it is thought to be a permanent therapeutic option (at least until a deeper understanding is found). Sticking with a medicine for life can be a challenge. First, it is common for people to experience treatment fatigue, when they tire of taking medicines for any number of reasons. There are also considerations of cost and the changing availability of product. If you can be flexible with your product choices during remission, you have the best chances of limiting boredom, having useful options on hand, and continuing treatment. And as you've read, there are many other positive health benefits of adding cannabis to your daily regimen.

+ **Dosing:** Cancer is terrifying and emotionally all-consuming, no matter at which stage you begin. The sooner the disease and symptoms can be treated, the better. For anyone who wants to begin this process and is new to cannabis, I typically recommend starting with moderate to high doses of CBD, on the order of 100–200 mg daily, preferably one to four times per day, as frequently as possible. Each day, the dose should either increase by about 5 to 10 percent, or an equivalent amount of a different cannabinoid should be added. When possible, THC should be added gradually, at increasing amounts, until you feel comfortable performing everyday tasks without impair. The ratios of euphoric and non-euphoric cannabinoids should be adjusted to your instinctual preference. In the setting of limited high-quality evidence-based research, I feel that it is still important to consider how my patients feel as a critical indicator of their well-being and the effectiveness of a cannabis regimen.

+ **Short-acting versus longer-lasting:** Any cannabis cancer treatment should be long-acting. If you are not experiencing sustained effects all day, you need to increase your dosage. The duration of each dose should be between six to eight hours. At three to four times a day, you should achieve complete coverage for every twenty-four-hour period. Don't wait until the effects completely wear off before you take the next dose. As time goes on, the doses will build on each other and you will become tolerant to their effects, even as they continue to battle against cancer and treat symptoms.

+ **Euphoric/non-euphoric:** The best available evidence points to better odds of success with high-dose, full-spectrum, terpene- and flavonoid-rich cannabis. The dosage advances that I recommend of THC sometimes create undesirable alterations of mood and mental state. For many who face a fast-approaching end, mental clarity and control may be both necessary and important. For those who want to curb the effects of THC, or who want to escalate doses on a faster timeline, add CBD to the mix in increasing amounts until you feel better.

+ **Compare products:** Compare the products containing specific terpenes and flavonoids to the master list in chapter one to make sure you are getting the benefits you are looking for. Some terpene components found in cannabis seem to enhance the effects of cannabinoids, and some terpenes are known to have cancer-fighting capabilities in their own right. These include linalool[10] and limonene.[11]

+ **Interactions with other medications:** The vast majority of my patients use cannabis as a cancer treatment along with traditional therapies. The consistent paradigm in medicine is that when you can hit a disease from multiple angles, you are going to get better results than any one treatment alone. However, when you're using cannabis, it's important to consider whether there might be a risk of making these traditional treatments less effective. Because of its ability to modulate immune function, it will interfere with some traditional cancer treatments like biologics, T-cell therapies, cancer vaccines, oncolytic virus therapy, and treatments that have immune-dependent effects such as doxorubicin and cisplatin, all of which otherwise have good, predictable outcomes. Discuss the benefits and concerns of bringing on cannabis with your oncologist. In some cases, using lower doses of cannabis for symptom management might be preferable to high-dose attempts at attacking cancer.

When You Cannot Access Legal THC

If you do not have access to a dispensary, you can purchase hemp or CBD-derived products online to treat cancer and its symptoms. The online marketplace offers versions of THC products that originated from CBD plants, which may be effective. You can purchase flower, concentrates, edibles, and tinctures that are analogous to THC products. You will need just as large volumes to maximize the likelihood of success. It appears that CBD products are less effective than THC but still likely more effective than not using them at all. Make sure to let your healthcare provider know that you are using high doses of CBD so that they can accurately monitor your health.

Consider Pretreating Cancer

The period between your cancer diagnosis and the start of your traditional treatment can act as an on-ramp for cannabis use. Proceeding slowly with increasing dosage is an easy way for someone to start becoming accustomed to the larger doses of cannabinoids that might have real, meaningful effects on cancers. It can also help your body adjust to potential side effects. For instance, my patient Mindy recently told me, "My chemo and radiation started on Wednesday, but since I've been taking cannabis for two weeks ahead of time, I feel less nauseous than I expected." A pretreating regimen can also stabilize your mood so that you can take in the information and instructions following your diagnosis, and it helps with the worry and anticipation of discomfort.

Pretreating with non-euphoric compounds, including CBD, CBDA, CBG, CBGA, CBC, and CBCA, is an accessible option in the online marketplace. This strategy will make the process of taking high-dose cannabinoids later more tolerable: beginning with the non-euphoric varieties may protect you from the cognitive impacts of high doses of THC that you will need later.

MEET THOMAS

Tom is one of my favorite patients, because he came to see me fully informed, and he did the work on his own to create remarkable results. This is his story in his own words:

> In 2014, my wife and I decided to buy property in rural Maine, where we could live off-grid and straighten out our lives. We went vegan and cleaned up our health by running and joining a gym. All was going great until 2019, when I was on my three-wheeler and I got into a crash. I punctured a lung and smashed ten ribs. We were so far out that I had to take myself to the hospital, but when I got there, I learned that my broken cage wasn't the worst of my problems. The doctors came in and told me that I had three tumors in my stomach and enlarged lymph nodes.

Long story short, my test results come back: I have something called follicular lymphoma, and besides the three cancerous tumors in my stomach, the cancer had moved into my bones.

In my earlier life I was a hospital pharmacy tech specialist and I prepared IVs for chemotherapy. It had been twenty years since I've worked in a pharmacy, but believe it or not, not a lot has changed. So, I have full knowledge what my treatment options were going to be. My wife and I decided to go to the best hospital near us, which was Dana-Farber in Boston, Massachusetts. When I got there, they said they were going to have to run me through six months of chemotherapy. They would hit me once a month with bendamustine plus rituximab, an immuno-chemotherapy and a regular chemo, for the rest of my life. They didn't know how fast the cancer was spreading or if the chemo would even work.

I had my first chemo treatment, and it was probably one of the scariest, most awful things I've ever been through. Nausea, vomiting, diarrhea. And bone pain: every single bone in my body was heaving with pain. The next time I went back, they adjusted my meds to include Zofran for the nausea. I ended up going to my second treatment; I wasn't adjusting at all. By the third treatment, I just was going downhill. I said to my wife, "I'm not going to make it through this. I've got to do something else."

I did a fair amount of research on my own. I couldn't sleep for quite some time, so I did a lot of reading. The research introduced me to cannabis, and I thought that I would give it a shot because there seems to be some real facts and some truth to it. I told the doctor who was administering the chemo that I was using cannabis. He was fine with it, although he suggested that I shouldn't smoke it, and try an edible form. I met Dr. Caplan, and I put in for my medical marijuana license.

I had messed around with pot as a kid, but never as a medicine. I read about Rick Simpson Oil (a type of full-spectrum cannabis oil) and what it does for people. I couldn't afford it, so I figured out how to make my own that would be as close to his formula. I started with 50 milligrams four to five times a day, and increased my dosage weekly by 25 to 50 milligrams, working my way up. Eventually, I made it up to 1,000 milligrams or a gram a day, which is a lot for anyone to manage. It took a good month to get up to the 1-gram dose. I'm not going to lie: it was actually tough to get up to that amount. I was taking 200 milligrams five times a day orally. I was making edibles, including cookies, and I learned how to put it in anything. I had to take time off work: you can't be eating a gram a day and going to work. And I tried a bunch of different strains, and found some that didn't affect me mentally. I learned about terpenes and worked with my dispensary to find plants that met my needs.

After about thirty days of getting up to close to a gram a day or 750 milligrams, I started to feel major changes. The stomach meds went away. They gave me tons of steroids that I would have to have that would last two to three days. I told them to kick back on that. At my next chemo infusion, I didn't have to take the Zofran and my appetite came back (I couldn't even taste food until I started using it) and my pain was managed. My anxiety was way less. I could sleep, and the ruminating thoughts about dying quieted down. My life kind of came back.

Once I was on cannabis, I was able to maintain my weight for the rest of my chemotherapy. Toward the end of my treatments, it just got easier and easier. The pain was gone. The bone pain was gone. I was feeling well enough that I could get back in my kayak, or try and ride my bike for a little while.

Then, amazingly, after the fourth month of treatment, my tumors were completely gone. I was in complete remission. I went through the next two cycles, complete remission. And then I had a one-year scan that just went by. I've been using cannabis as a medicine now not as strong. You don't need that amount. So, I would do maybe 100 milligrams a day, which is what I call my maintenance dose. And after two years, I'm still totally cancer-free. I'm back to riding my bike two hundred miles a week, feeling great.

Making the Right Decision for You

If you are looking for additional treatments to cancer, you are already at the cutting edge of science. Without good data, I know this decision can be daunting. However, the risk-to-benefit analysis of including cannabis to me is pretty clear: cannabis is not going to make your cancer worse. And you have the potential to feel much better.

What's more, cannabis can offer a renewed sense of optimism. I can't tell you how many people come to me with Stage 4 cancers, thinking about dying. And then when I raise the possibility that their cancer may retreat, the common response I hear is, "Wow, I was not prepared for that. Nobody has ever given me any hope."

It's important to acknowledge, however, that the people who return to me, over the course of their cancer treatment and cannabis consumption, are the patients who have survived. There have been many memorable and heart-wrenching occasions when I have discovered that a patient of mine succumbed to their cancer. Despite earnest efforts, I have not been able to discern the complete set of qualities of those patients who thrive from those who do not.

Whether their fate was driven more by biology, environmental factors, or just time remains a mystery. Even with these unknowns and losses, if it were me or a loved one facing a diagnosis of cancer, I can assure you that cannabis would undoubtedly be part of the treatment journey.

CHAPTER 16

Creating an End-of-Life Plan

The very last aspect of a family medicine practice is *palliative care*, where the goal is to alleviate suffering and improve the quality of life for patients with serious illness. Often, these are patients with cancer, advanced heart failure, or neurodegenerative diseases like Alzheimer's disease and dementia. Occasionally, palliative care addresses the needs of people who are not dying yet are struggling to get relief from their hard-to-treat chronic illnesses. They are largely uncomfortable, understandably upset, and deeply unhappy. Yet when they start using cannabis products, I see their mood shift. They become content, lively, and happy, even when they know they are confronting terrible challenges, including mortality.

End-of-life care is a section of medicine where we have the opportunity to use all of the tools available, even the ones that are less rigorously studied, if there is the potential to help someone. So even with a limited amount of "gold standard" scientific studies, I feel comfortable prescribing cannabis to these patients. I strongly believe that people deserve to die with dignity, which means that there is no reason to be uncomfortable during the last phase of life. It is dreadful to witness someone at the end of their days trapped in pain, sleeplessness, anxiety, and sorrow. In contrast, it is heartwarming to share the final days of someone's life, reminiscing about their most joyful moments and fond memories. To my mind, a dignified death also means that the person has the ability to be focused in the present moment and at peace, without being depressed or anxious. With a clear head, these individuals are often able to achieve a deeply positive self-reflection.

Very often, it's not the person who is dying who reaches out to me: it's a family member. Their loved one may be in the hospital, has been given a terminal diagnosis, and they want to make that person as comfortable as possible. Sometimes, the patient has been given hospice orders (meaning pain medications and morphine), yet family members don't want their loved one to be drugged out or die in their sleep because they can't breathe. Not surprisingly, they also want to talk about which cannabis products are appropriate for themselves so that they can cope with their inevitable loss better. It's normal for extreme stressors like death to compel people to increase their focus on self-care. What's more, many of these people who approach cannabis at this time find that it addresses other aspects of their health as well.

Decisions for End-of-Life Care

If you or a loved one has received a terminal diagnosis, or you're living with a chronic condition, you have the unique opportunity to decide what the end can look like. Each of the following decisions can be augmented with an effective cannabis therapy:

+ **Goals of care:** Consider what a good death looks like. I often hear from my patients that they desire symptom management, avoidance of suffering, and the ability to maintain a clear decision-making process, including choices for nonessential medications, resuscitation directives, and feeding instructions. They want to have control over their waking and sleeping hours, and they want to minimize interruptions by medical staff administering tests and medicines. In order to meet these needs, I always recommend that you explore your cannabis options early. Think about how you want to feel, how compatible those feelings are with your goals of care, and then find the product of choice that you can then calibrate when you really need it. Experiment with a wide scope of choices. One of the most common mistakes that people make with cannabis therapies is not appreciating that it takes time to find your optimal dose. The more time that you can give to exploring cannabis early on, the less time you'll need later to feel comfortable.

+ **Choosing your preferred location:** I have found that most people would prefer to die at home, surrounded by familiarities and loved ones, although many do not manage to do so. If this is something you desire, make sure that your home is well equipped ahead of time: You may require a hospital bed to make the positioning associated with sleeping, eating, and wakeful life easier to manage. You will want systems to organize medications, routines, and convenient alarms to help automate these regimens. If you prefer a hospital or hospice setting, it is also worth careful planning ahead of time. Since the passage of the Right to Try Act of 2018, palliative care programs in the United States are empowered to facilitate the use of cannabis for all patients. Nonetheless, it is still critical to understand the matching process with how cannabis works for each individual, and to enable the palliative care team to use this knowledge effectively.

+ **Cultural and religious traditions:** Throughout history, cannabis has been continuously used by a wide variety of faiths for sacramental connection between religious leaders, their followers, and the divine. This practice offers the opportunity to connect individuals to their own deep spiritual queries. In the face of death, we know that many turn to religion for comfort, so it is no surprise that cannabis can help facilitate and even augment the same power of spiritual review.

+ **Communicating thoughtfully and accurately:** It's very difficult to hear and fully understand bad news. Cannabis can help us calm down and focus so that we can identify and express our true goals of care and our personal preferences for end of life, and to appoint surrogate decision-makers within the family or close friends. Although many people have the impression that cannabis impairs or distracts from normal thought or communication, the reality is quite the opposite. Cannabis quiets distractions so that you have a more open awareness to consider and communicate your choices.

+ **Care coordination:** The reality of hospital and nursing home medicine is that within many understaffed, underfunded facilities, patients at the end of life are frequently left alone, disconnected from their families. Patients can also feel bewildered because daytime and nighttime blur together, as hospital staff checks them intermittently at all hours of the day and night. Cannabis can help regulate your internal clock so that you sleep at night and are awake and alert during the day. And by allowing you to focus and remain calm and comfortable, you will be better able to understand, and even participate in, transfers between healthcare settings.

Expecting and Treating Symptoms

Patients in the advanced stages of a life-threatening illness typically experience multiple symptoms, often resulting from a number of factors, including the specific disease, from treatments, from other conditions, or from medications.[1] Because cannabis works on a multi-system level, one therapy can address many complaints at the same time, and cannabis seems to be compatible with most modern medicines.

We've learned from end-of-life cannabis consumption that people wished they'd tried these options sooner. The prevalence of pain among patients with terminal illnesses is particularly high,[2] and as you've learned, cannabis addresses pain extremely well. Cannabis is an ideal pain reliever for the wide variety of symptoms people have at end of life. And there are so many ways of delivering the necessary cannabinoids. For example, if you can't swallow, there are patches, suppositories, nose drops, or lotions.

Recommendations for end-stage patients are tailored to specific aims and conditions. For some patients, lucid pain relief is a priority, while others want to combat depression or anxiety. In instances where there are multiple interacting illnesses, cannabis products can deal with symptoms quicker than traditional pharmaceuticals, without the lingering effects that can interfere with other assessments and treatments. Generally, more powerful dosages that are of short duration are preferable. Sample regimens for each of these have been listed previously in this book.

The most common symptoms are:

+ Anorexia/lack of appetite/weight loss
+ Anticipatory grief
+ Anxiety
+ Confusion/delirium
+ Constipation
+ Cough
+ Depression
+ Diarrhea
+ Dysphagia (difficulty swallowing)
+ Dyspnea (shortness of breath/breathlessness)
+ Edema (swelling, particularly in the arms and legs)
+ Fatigue
+ Hopelessness/demoralization
+ Insomnia
+ Nausea (with or without vomiting)
+ Pain
+ Xerostomia (dry mouth)

Adjusting to a Better Diurnal Rhythm

Many people at end of life lose their ability for diurnal regulation—staying awake during the day and sleeping at night—particularly when they are in hospitals. It's not surprising: when you're in pain or uncomfortable, you're up all night, anyway. In hospitals, the constant light in the hallways and nighttime interruptions compound the problem.

One of the known benefits of cannabis therapy is that the specific options discussed throughout the book that are better for sleep (calming), or for increasing energy (activating), can be used to help people become comfortable at the end of life. Having those options at the ready can vastly improve sleepiness or wakefulness.

Products for Hospice Care

The medications often prescribed during hospice care—sedatives and opiates—are frequently overpowering, leaving the patient numb and altering perception and personality in extreme ways. Morphine offers complete relief from pain, yet when people take it, there are slowing effects on the breathing centers of the brain, and someone taking it may be unable to communicate serious issues. Cannabis solves the pain problem without affecting normal breathing, and at the same time, it allows the person to engage in social relationships.

Sedatives like benzodiazepines (Klonopin, Xanax, Ativan, Valium) will make one feel extremely sleepy, sometimes to the point of unconsciousness. When they are awake, they will feel loopy and be incoherent. This leaves the dying person feeling disconnected from reality during their last opportunities to engage with family and friends.

I have had several patients who began their exploration with cannabis when they were looking for a clearheaded alternative to the end-of-life pain relief that sedatives and opiates offer. Their families were grateful that cannabis allowed their loved one gifts beyond measure: the dignity and the ability to interact with others, and at the same time, to alleviate their pain. I have also had family members connect with me during the first few days of cannabis therapy to let me know that their parent is back from death's door, even though they are still in the process of dying. Some of the most common suggestions for cannabis products that replace morphine and sedatives include:

+ Long-lasting high-THC choices (chocolate, gummies)
+ Short-acting low-dose THC choices (tincture, dissolving tablet, inhaled cannabis)
+ Regular medium-dosed CBD, microdosed throughout the day
+ Mixed THC and CBD with therapeutic additives (melatonin, caffeine, lavender, etc.)
+ For those who can't swallow, consider suppositories and/or misting via nebulization

The Last Hours of Life

Cannabis can make end of life more comfortable, and it may prolong the course. For example, if appetite diminishes at end of life, and you use cannabis to stimulate appetite, that, in some degree, extends one's timeline. We also know that prolonging joy, comfort, pleasure, and contentment with cannabis can make one more hesitant to want to die.

Cannabis cannot be used as a tool to hasten death. There's no amount of cannabis that someone could reasonably consume that would be toxic. That being said, the medicines that are available to help end someone's life are sometimes unpleasant, and combining them with cannabis can ease discomfort and fear of the unknown.

Many people at the end of their life have very precarious heart conditions. In this one instance, cannabis does pose a potential concern, because of its direct stimulating effect on the heart. For this reason, approach this delicate circumstance with medical guidance that will meet your specific concerns with appropriate, individualized care.

In the very last hours of life, people will experience a set of symptoms that is very predictable. Cannabis might hasten the sequence of events a little bit, but at the same time the loved one isn't suffering. Symptoms to watch for include:

+ Convulsions
+ Death rattle: gurgling or crackling sounds
+ Decreased level of consciousness
+ Decreased urine output
+ Difficulty swallowing liquids
+ Loss of skin color in extremities

MEET GIGI

My patient Gigi recently passed from metastatic cancer. She knew the end was near and wanted to share a lucid day with her family at her bedside.

The opiates she had been prescribed made her foggy and tired, and they left her generally feeling unlike herself. Cannabis, on the other hand, helped her experience levity and comfort at the end, and gave the family lasting memories of a joyful woman who still had to travel the most difficult road.

After she passed, her son Tom told me, "Your advice to my family has been a tremendous gift. Mom's last days were comfortable, fantastic, and full of laughter. We were telling jokes and reminiscing. Instead of her moaning in bed all the time, she was present and communicating. I couldn't have asked for a better end for a more deserving woman."

Afterword: Achieving the Best of Health and Happiness

Ultimately, what is exceptional about cannabis is the opportunity to capture a dose of joy in the face of adversity. I believe that we each have the opportunity, if not the incentive, to make every day matter. As you've read throughout this book, my hope is that you have found many ways that cannabis can serve as an effective treatment to make every day better, by alleviating discomfort and magnifying well-being.

You now have the instructions to build your own tool kit, not only to treat the ailments you may be experiencing, but to improve your day-to-day life. Every day doesn't have to be a stressful grind. And even in sickness, you can have some amount of respite. Whenever you are uncomfortable, you now have the choice and power to dispense doses of joy and relaxation. Sometimes, that small amount of joy is the difference between surviving and thriving.

We live in a world that often feels like we are navigating our health dramas alone. The existing, traditional medical infrastructure is built on the assumption that people don't change much, and that the appropriate medication is always available, affordable, and consistent. This outlook is flawed and is not in alignment with the realities of life. So, first and foremost, I want to invite you into the broader community of cannabis medicine, where you will no longer feel like you are alone. In spite of a steady battle against social and political hardship for generations, the cannabis community, including the millions of people who consume cannabis to ease suffering, is warm, joyful, and welcoming.

I also want you to remember that cannabis products operate within a marketplace that is always changing, adapting, and improving. This is important, because despite what may be easier to believe, there is no state of "normal" either in the marketplace or in your own life. The world is ever-changing. Your mind and body change over time naturally, and when you have cannabis on board, the change may be dramatic. When it comes to the cannabis marketplace, which is just in its infancy, the only thing I can guarantee is that it will also be changing: the product you enjoyed yesterday may no longer be available the next time you shop. Even if it is, the product you enjoyed on what you thought was one of your "good days" may not work as well when you are having a really bad day. Keep trying new products, new dosages, and new frequencies so that you will have a full complement of options for when you need them.

So, on this journey, try to keep an open mind. There will be new products that are waiting to be tried and may bring even more relief. What's more, have the courage to remember that you know yourself. You are the master of your fate. The more agency you have, and the more empowered you feel by learning about your health options and your personal evolution, the better you will feel.

Recommended Reading

Sociopolitical History of Cannabis

Corva, Dominic, and Joshua S. Meisel. *The Routledge Handbook of Post-Prohibition Cannabis Research*. Routledge, 2021.

Duvall, Chris S. *The African Roots of Marijuana*. Duke University Press, 2019.

Grinspoon, Peter. *Seeing Through the Smoke: A Cannabis Specialist Untangles the Truth About Marijuana*. Prometheus, 2023.

Herer, Jack. *The Emperor Wears No Clothes: A History of Cannabis/Hemp/Marijuana*, 14th edition. Self-published, 2020.

EMCDDA Monographs: *A Cannabis Reader: Global Issues and Local Experiences* (a free resource: https://www.emcdda.europa.eu/publications/monographs/cannabis-volume1_en).

Scientific Analysis of Cannabis Chemistry

Iversen, Leslie. *The Science of Marijuana*, 3rd edition. Oxford University Press, 2018.

Montoya, Ivan D., and Susan R. B. Weiss. *Cannabis Use Disorders*. Springer, 2019.

Thomas, Brian F., and Mahmoud A. ElSohly. *The Analytical Chemistry of Cannabis: Quality Assessment, Assurance, and Regulation of Medicinal Marijuana and Cannabinoid Preparations*. Elsevier, 2015.

Cooking with Cannabis

Hua, Stephanie. *Edibles: Small Bites for the Modern Cannabis Kitchen*. Chronicle
    Books, 2018.

Wolf, Laurie, and Mary Thigpen. *Marijuana Edibles: 40 Easy and Delicious
    Cannabis-Infused Desserts*. Alpha, 2016.

Growing Cannabis

Cervantes, Jorge. *Marijuana Grow Basics: The Easy Guide for Cannabis Aficionados*.
    Van Patten Publishing, 2009.

Thomas, Mel. *Cannabis Cultivation: A Complete Grower's Guide*, 3rd edition.
    Green Candy Press, 2012.

Acknowledgments

Thank you to all of my patients who have allowed me to support them and learn from their cannabis therapeutic journeys. My protocols for effective cannabis care are directly influenced by their knowledge and experience.

A special thanks to Lokesh Chugh; Peter Grinspoon, MD; Howard Kessler; Sean Collins; Dave Batista; Kristen Rafuse; Camila O'Brien; and my medical colleagues and mentors, who have each inspired me to see, learn, and grow from a wide array of professional viewpoints.

I would like to acknowledge my better half and brilliant wife, Erin Caplan, NP, for her patience and love, and with whom I have found peace, ready to take on the world! Along with my bride, I am grateful to my enormous family, including my parents, Dr. Louis Caplan, MD, and Brenda Caplan; Laura Greer, LCSW-C, and Daniel Greer; Jonathan Caplan and Patricia Caplan; David Caplan, Esq., and Denys Caplan; Jeremy and Caren Caplan; and my aunt, Gloria Sterling, PhD, as well as my four children, Lola, Audrey, Sebastian, and Theodore. It is thanks to this circus of personality and knowledge that I have learned to question with equanimity, challenge with respect, and know when to live, love, and let live.

Thank you, Pam Liflander, for helping me put my thoughts on these pages. My agent, Carol Mann, introduced me to the brilliant team at BenBella, including Claire Schulz, Sarah Avinger, and Leah Wilson. Thanks to all for helping me share my knowledge with the world.

Notes

Introduction

1. Han BH, Palamar JJ. Trends in cannabis use among older adults in the United States, 2015–2018. *JAMA Intern Med.* 2020;180(4):609–611. doi:10.1001/jamainternmed.2019.7517.

Chapter 1

1. Mihai A. Humans started growing cannabis 12,000 years ago—for food, fibers, and probably to get high. ZME Science, July 19, 2021. https://www.zmescience.com/science/archaeology/humans-started-growing-cannabis-12000-years-ago-for-food-fibers-and-probably-to-get-high/.
2. Zuardi AW. History of cannabis as a medicine: a review. *Braz J Psychiatry.* 2006 Jun;28(2):153–57. doi: 10.1590/s1516-44462006000200015. Epub 2006 Jun 26. PMID: 16810401.
3. Vago R, et al. The Mediterranean diet as a source of bioactive molecules with cannabinomimetic activity in prevention and therapy strategy. *Nutrients.* 2022 Jan 21;14(3):468. doi: 10.3390/nu14030468. PMID: 35276827; PMCID: PMC8839035.

Chapter 2

1. Mikuriya TH. Marijuana in medicine: past, present and future. *Calif Med.* 1969;110:34–40.

2. Zuardi AW. History of cannabis as a medicine: a review. *Braz J Psychiatry*. 2006 Jun;28(2):153–7. doi: 10.1590/s1516-44462006000200015. Epub 2006 Jun 26. PMID: 16810401.

3. Sample I. Scientists find genetic mutation that makes woman feel no pain. *The Guardian*, March 27, 2019. https://www.theguardian.com/science/2019/mar/28 /scientists-find-genetic-mutation-that-makes-woman-feel-no-pain.

4. Panossian A. Understanding adaptogenic activity: Specificity of the pharmacological action of adaptogens and other phytochemicals. *Annals of the New York Academy of Sciences*. 2017 Aug;1401(1):49–64. Epub 2017 Jun 22.

Chapter 3

1. Libzon S, Schleider LB, Saban N, Levit L, Tamari Y, Linder I, Lerman-Sagie T, Blumkin L. Medical cannabis for pediatric moderate to severe complex motor disorders. *J Child Neurol*. 2018 Aug;33(9):565–571. doi: 10.1177/0883073818773028. Epub 2018 May 16. PMID: 29766748.

Chapter 5

1. U.S. Department of Agriculture and U.S. Department of Health and Human Services. *Dietary guidelines for Americans, 2020–2025*. 9th edition. December 2020.

2. Rossi F, Punzo F, Umano GR, Argenziano M, Miraglia Del Giudice E. Role of cannabinoids in obesity. *Int J Mol Sci*. 2018 Sep 10;19(9):2690. doi: 10.3390 /ijms19092690. PMID: 30201891; PMCID: PMC6163475.

3. Sihag J, Di Marzo V. (Wh)olistic (E)ndocannabinoidome-Microbiome-Axis Modulation through (N)utrition (WHEN) to curb obesity and related disorders. *Lipids Health Dis*. 2022 Jan 14;21(1):9. doi: 10.1186/s12944-021-01609-3. PMID: 35027074; PMCID: PMC8759188.

Chapter 6

1. Marco EM, Laviola G. The endocannabinoid system in the regulation of emotions throughout lifespan: a discussion on therapeutic perspectives. *J Psychopharmacol*. 2012 Jan;26(1):150–63. doi: 10.1177/0269881111408459. Epub 2011 Jun 21. PMID: 21693551.

2. Bitencourt RM, Pamplona FA, Takahashi RN. Facilitation of contextual fear memory extinction and anti-anxiogenic effects of AM404 and cannabidiol in conditioned rats. *Eur Neuropsychopharmacol*. 2018;18:849–859.

3. O'Sullivan SE, Kendall PJ, and Kendall DA. Endocannabinoids and the cardio-vascular response to stress. *J Psychopharmacol*. 2012;26:71–82.

4. Kohler O, Krogh J, Mors O, and Benros ME. Inflammation in depression and the potential for anti-inflammatory treatment. Current neuropharmacology. 2016;14(7):732–742. https://doi.org/10.2174/1570159x14666151208113700.

5. Ranganathan M, Braley G, Pittman B, Cooper T, Perry E, Krystal J, D'Souza DC. The effects of cannabinoids on serum cortisol and prolactin in humans. *Psychopharmacology (Berl)*. 2009 May;203(4):737–44. doi: 10.1007/s00213-008-1422-2. Epub 2008 Dec 16. PMID: 19083209; PMCID: PMC2863108.

6. NIDA. 2021, April 13. How does marijuana produce its effects? Retrieved from https://nida.nih.gov/publications/research-reports/marijuana/how-does-marijuana-produce-its-effects on 2022, May 23

Chapter 7

1. Nedeltcheva AV, Scheer FAJL. Metabolic effects of sleep disruption, links to obesity and diabetes. *Current Opinion in Endocrinology & Diabetes and Obesity*. 2014;21(4):293–298. doi:10.1097/med.0000000000000082.

2. Weich S, Pearce HL, Croft P, Singh S, Crome I, Bashford J, Frisher M. Effect of anxiolytic and hypnotic drug prescriptions on mortality hazards: retrospective cohort study. *BMJ*. 2014 Mar 19;348:g1996. doi: 10.1136/bmj.g1996. PMID: 24647164; PMCID: PMC3959619.

3. Arble DM, Bass J, Behn CD, Butler MP, Challet E, Czeisler C, Depner CM, Elmquist J, Franken P, Grandner MA, Hanlon EC, Keene AC, Joyner MJ, Karatsoreos I, Kern PA, Klein S, Morris CJ, Pack AI, Panda S, Ptacek LJ, Punjabi NM, Sassone-Corsi P, Scheer FA, Saxena R, Seaquest ER, Thimgan MS, Van Cauter E, Wright KP. Impact of sleep and circadian disruption on energy balance and diabetes: A summary of workshop discussions. *Sleep*. 2015 Dec 1;38(12):1849–60. doi: 10.5665/sleep.5226. PMID: 26564131; PMCID: PMC4667373.

4. Lafaye G, Desterke C, Marulaz L, Benyamina A. Cannabidiol affects cir-cadian clock core complex and its regulation in microglia cells. *Addict Biol*. 2019 Sep;24(5):921–934. doi: 10.1111/adb.12660. Epub 2018 Oct 11. PMID: 30307084.

5. Patricelli MP, Patterson JE, Boger DL, Cravatt BF. An endogenous sleep-inducing compound is a novel competitive inhibitor of fatty acid amide hydrolase. *Bioorg Med Chem Lett*. 1998 Mar 17;8(6):613-8. doi: 10.1016/s0960-894x(98)00073-0. PMID: 9871570.

Chapter 8

1. Ramachandran R. Neurogenic inflammation and its role in migraine. *Semin Immunopathol.* 2018 May;40(3):301–314. doi: 10.1007/s00281-018-0676-y. Epub 2018 Mar 22. PMID: 29568973.

2. Leimuranta P, Khiroug L, Giniatullin R. Emerging role of (endo)cannabinoids in migraine. *Front Pharmacol.* 2018 Apr 24;9:420. doi: 10.3389 /fphar.2018.00420. PMID: 29740328; PMCID: PMC5928495.

3. Park SN, Lim YK, Freire MO, Cho E, Jin D, Kook JK. Antimicrobial effect of linalool and α-terpineol against periodontopathic and cariogenic bacteria. *Anaerobe.* 2012 Jun;18(3):369–72. doi: 10.1016/j.anaerobe.2012.04.001. Epub 2012 Apr 17. PMID: 22537719.

Chapter 9

1. Stefano GB, Liu Y, Goligorsky M. Cannabinoid receptors are coupled to nitric oxide release in invertebrate immunocytes, microglia, and human monocytes. *Journal of Biological Chemistry.* 1996;271(32):19238–19242. doi:10.1074/jbc.271.32.19238.

2. D'Souza DC, Pittman B, Perry E, Simen A. Preliminary evidence of cannabinoid effects on brain-derived neurotrophic factor (BDNF) levels in humans. *Psychopharmacology (Berl).* 2009 Mar;202(4):569–78. doi: 10.1007/s00213-008 -1333-2. Epub 2008 Sep 21. PMID: 18807247; PMCID: PMC2791800.

3. Arévalo-Martín A, García-Ovejero D, Gómez O, Rubio-Araiz A, Navarro-Galve B, Guaza C, Molina-Holgado E, Molina-Holgado F. CB2 cannabinoid receptors as an emerging target for demyelinating diseases: from neuroimmune interactions to cell replacement strategies. *Br J Pharmacol.* 2008 Jan;153(2):216–25. doi: 10.1038/sj.bjp.0707466. Epub 2007 Sep 24. PMID: 17891163; PMCID: PMC2219542.

4. Deurveilher S, Golovin T, Hall S, Semba K. Microglia dynamics in sleep/wake states and in response to sleep loss. *Neurochem Int.* 2021 Feb;143:104944. doi: 10.1016/j.neuint.2020.104944. Epub 2020 Dec 23. PMID: 33359188.

5. Stowell RD, Sipe GO, Dawes RP, Batchelor HN, Lordy KA, Whitelaw BS, Stoessel MB, Bidlack JM, Brown E, Sur M, Majewska AK. Noradrenergic signaling in the wakeful state inhibits microglial surveillance and synaptic plasticity in the mouse visual cortex. *Nat Neurosci.* 2019 Nov;22(11):1782–1792. doi: 10.1038/s41593-019-0514-0. Epub 2019 Oct 21. Erratum in: *Nat Neurosci.* 2020 Jan;23(1):152. PMID: 31636451; PMCID: PMC6875777.

6. Sommerlad A, Sabia S, Singh-Manoux A, Lewis G, Livingston G. Association of social contact with dementia and cognition: 28-year follow-up of the Whitehall II cohort study. *PLoS Med.* 2019 Aug 2;16(8):e1002862. doi: 10.1371/journal .pmed.1002862. PMID: 31374073; PMCID: PMC6677303.

7. Root M, Ravine E, Harper A. Flavonol intake and cognitive decline in middle-aged adults. *J Med Food.* 2015 Dec;18(12):1327–32. doi: 10.1089/jmf.2015.0010. Epub 2015 Sep 1. PMID: 26325006.

8. Gęgotek A, Atalay S, Rogowska-Wrzesińska A, Skrzydlewska E. The effect of cannabidiol on UV-induced changes in intracellular signaling of 3D-cultured skin keratinocytes. *Int J Mol Sci.* 2021 Feb 2;22(3):1501. doi: 10.3390/ijms 22031501. PMID: 33540902; PMCID: PMC7867360.

9. Raja A, Ahmadi S, de Costa F, Li N, Kerman K. Attenuation of oxidative stress by cannabinoids and cannabis extracts in differentiated neuronal cells. *Pharmaceuticals (Basel).* 2020 Oct 22;13(11):328. doi: 10.3390/ph13110328. PMID: 33105840; PMCID: PMC7690570.

10. Vitanova KS, Stringer KM, Benitez DP, Brenton J, Cummings DM. Dementia associated with disorders of the basal ganglia. *J Neurosci Res.* 2019 Dec;97(12):1728–1741. doi: 10.1002/jnr.24508. Epub 2019 Aug 7. PMID: 31392765.

11. García C, Palomo-Garo C, Gómez-Gálvez Y, Fernández-Ruiz J. Cannabinoid-dopamine interactions in the physiology and physiopathology of the basal ganglia. *Br J Pharmacol.* 2016 Jul;173(13):2069–79. doi: 10.1111/bph.13215. Epub 2015 Jul 31. PMID: 26059564; PMCID: PMC4908199.

12. Szutorisz H, Hurd YL. Epigenetic effects of cannabis exposure. *Biol Psychiatry.* 2016 Apr 1;79(7):586–94. doi: 10.1016/j.biopsych.2015.09.014. Epub 2015 Nov 3. PMID: 26546076; PMCID: PMC4789113.

13. Esposito G, Scuderi C, Valenza M, Togna GI, Latina V, De Filippis D, Cipriano M, Carratù MR, Iuvone T, Steardo L. Cannabidiol reduces Aβ-induced neuroinflammation and promotes hippocampal neurogenesis through PPARγ involvement. *PLoS One.* 2011;6(12):e28668. doi: 10.1371/journal.pone.0028668. Epub 2011 Dec 5. PMID: 22163051; PMCID: PMC3230631.

14. Schuele LL, Schuermann B, Bilkei-Gorzo A, Gorgzadeh S, Zimmer A, Leidmaa E. Regulation of adult neurogenesis by the endocannabinoid-producing enzyme diacylglycerol lipase alpha (DAGLa). *Sci Rep.* 2022 Jan 12;12(1):633. doi: 10.1038/s41598-021-04600-1. PMID: 35022487; PMCID: PMC8755832.

15. Campos AC, Ortega Z, Palazuelos J, Fogaça MV, Aguiar DC, Díaz-Alonso J, Ortega-Gutiérrez S, Vázquez-Villa H, Moreira FA, Guzmán M, Galve-Roperh I, Guimarães FS. The anxiolytic effect of cannabidiol on chronically stressed mice depends on hippocampal neurogenesis: involvement of the endocannabinoid

system. *Int J Neuropsychopharmacol.* 2013 Jul;16(6):1407–19. doi: 10.1017 /S1461145712001502. Epub 2013 Jan 9. PMID: 23298518.

16. Katz I, Katz D, Shoenfeld Y, Porat-Katz BS. Clinical Evidence for Utilizing Cannabinoids in the Elderly. *Isr Med Assoc J.* 2017 Feb;19(2):71–75. PMID: 28457053.

17. Suliman NA, Taib CNM, Moklas MAM, Basir R. Delta-9-tetrahydrocannabinol (Δ9-THC) induce neurogenesis and improve cognitive performances of male Sprague Dawley rats. *Neurotox Res.* 2018 Feb;33(2):402–411. doi: 10.1007/s12640-017-9806-x. Epub 2017 Sep 21. PMID: 28933048; PMCID: PMC5766723.

18. Fernández-Ruiz J, Romero J, Ramos JA. Endocannabinoids and neurodegenerative disorders: Parkinson's disease, Huntington's chorea, Alzheimer's disease, and others. *Handb Exp Pharmacol.* 2015;231:233–59. doi: 10.1007/978-3-319 -20825-1_8. PMID: 26408163.

19. Woodward MR, Harper DG, Stolyar A, Forester BP, Ellison JM. Dronabinol for the treatment of agitation and aggressive behavior in acutely hospitalized severely demented patients with noncognitive behavioral symptoms. Am J Geriatr Psychiatry. 2014 Apr;22(4):415–9. doi: 10.1016/j.jagp.2012.11.022. Epub 2013 Apr 15. PMID: 23597932.

20. Foebel A, Ballokova A, Wellens NI, Fialova D, Milisen K, Liperoti R, Hirdes JP. A retrospective, longitudinal study of factors associated with new antipsychotic medication use among recently admitted long-term care residents. *BMC Geriatr.* 2015 Oct 19;15:128. doi: 10.1186/s12877-015-0127-8. PMID: 26482028; PMCID: PMC4615888.

21. Martorell AJ, Paulson AL, Suk HJ, Abdurrob F, Drummond GT, Guan W, Young JZ, Kim DN, Kritskiy O, Barker SJ, Mangena V, Prince SM, Brown EN, Chung K, Boyden ES, Singer AC, Tsai LH. Multi-sensory gamma stimulation ameliorates Alzheimer's-associated pathology and improves cognition. *Cell.* 2019 Apr 4;177(2):256–271.e22. doi: 10.1016/j.cell.2019.02.014. Epub 2019 Mar 14. PMID: 30879788; PMCID: PMC6774262.

22. Oleson EB, Cheer JF. A brain on cannabinoids: the role of dopamine release in reward seeking. *Cold Spring Harb Perspect Med.* 2012 Aug 1;2(8):a012229. doi: 10.1101/cshperspect.a012229. PMID: 22908200; PMCID: PMC3405830.

23. Stampanoni Bassi M, Sancesario A, Morace R, Centonze D, Iezzi E. Cannabinoids in Parkinson's Disease. *Cannabis Cannabinoid Res.* 2017 Feb 1;2(1):21–29. doi: 10.1089/can.2017.0002. PMID: 28861502; PMCID: PMC5436333.

24. García C, Palomo-Garo C, Gómez-Gálvez Y, Fernández-Ruiz J. Cannabinoid-dopamine interactions in the physiology and physiopathology of the basal

ganglia. *Br J Pharmacol.* 2016 Jul;173(13):2069–79. doi: 10.1111/bph.13215. Epub 2015 Jul 31. PMID: 26059564; PMCID: PMC4908199.

Chapter 10

1. Zaheer S, Kumar D, Khan MT, Giyanwani PR, Kiran F. Epilepsy and cannabis: a literature review. *Cureus.* 2018 Sep 10;10(9):e3278. doi: 10.7759 /cureus.3278. PMID: 30443449; PMCID: PMC6235654.
2. Easterford K, Clough P, Comish S, Lawton L, Duncan S. The use of complementary medicines and alternative practitioners in a cohort of patients with epilepsy. *Epilepsy Behav.* 2005 Feb;6(1):59–62. doi: 10.1016/j.yebeh.2004.10.007. PMID: 15652735.
3. O'Shaughnessy WB. On the preparations of the Indian hemp, or gunjah: cannabis indica their effects on the animal system in health, and their utility in the treatment of tetanus and other convulsive diseases. *Prov Med J Retrosp Med Sci.* 1843;5:363–9.
4. Stempel AV, Stumpf A, Zhang HY, Özdoğan T, Pannasch U, Theis AK, Otte DM, Wojtalla A, Rácz I, Ponomarenko A, Xi ZX, Zimmer A, Schmitz D. Cannabinoid type 2 receptors mediate a cell type-specific plasticity in the hippocampus. *Neuron.* 2016 May 18;90(4):795–809. doi: 10.1016/j.neuron.2016.03.034. Epub 2016 Apr 28. PMID: 27133464; PMCID: PMC5533103.
5. Federation Proceedings, Federation of American Society for Experimental Biology, vol. 8, lY49:284.
6. Consroe PF, Wood GC, Buchsbaum H. Anticonvulsant nature of marihuana smoking. *JAMA.* 1975;234(3):306–307. doi:10.1001/jama.1975.03260 160054015.
7. Gross DW, Hamm J, Ashworth NL, Quigley D. Marijuana use and epilepsy: prevalence in patients of a tertiary care epilepsy center. *Neurology.* 2004 Jun 8;62(11):2095–7. doi: 10.1212/01.wnl.0000127623.03766.75. PMID: 15184622.

Chapter 11

1. Parmar N, Ho WS. N-arachidonoyl glycine, an endogenous lipid that acts as a vasorelaxant via nitric oxide and large conductance calcium-activated potassium channels. *Br J Pharmacol.* 2010 Jun;160(3):594–603. doi: 10.1111/j.1476-5381 .2009.00622.x. Epub 2010 Feb 5. PMID: 20136843; PMCID: PMC2931560.
2. Horvath G, Kekesi G, Nagy E, Benedek G. The role of TRPV1 receptors in the antinociceptive effect of anandamide at spinal level. *Pain.* 2008;134:277–284. doi: 10.1016/j.pain.2007.04.032.

3. Vučković S, Srebro D, Vujović KS, Vučetić Č, Prostran M. Cannabinoids and pain: new insights from old molecules. *Front. Pharmacol.* 2018;9:1259. doi: 10.3389/fphar.2018.01259

4. Mack A, Joy J. Marijuana as medicine? The science beyond the controversy. Washington, DC. National Academies Press (US); 2000. 7, MARIJUANA AND MUSCLE SPASTICITY. https://www.ncbi.nlm.nih.gov/books/NBK224382/.

5. Hohmann AG. Targeting CB2 receptors and the endocannabinoid system for the treatment of pain. *Brain Res. Rev.* 2009;60:255–266. doi: 10.1016/j.brainresrev.2008.12.003.

6. Rodrigues RS, Lourenço DM, Paulo SL, Mateus JM, Ferreira MF, Mouro FM, Moreira JB, Ribeiro FF, Sebastião AM, Xapelli S. Cannabinoid actions on neural stem cells: implications for pathophysiology. *Molecules.* 2019 Apr 5;24(7):1350. doi: 10.3390/molecules24071350. PMID: 30959794; PMCID: PMC6480122.

7. Miller H, De Leo N, Badach J, Lin A, Williamson J, Bonawitz S, Ostrovsky O. Role of marijuana components on the regenerative ability of stem cells. *Cell Biochem Funct.* 2021 Apr;39(3):432–441. doi: 10.1002/cbf.3609. Epub 2020 Dec 21. PMID: 33349985.

8. Miller H, De Leo N, Badach J, Lin A, Williamson J, Bonawitz S, Ostrovsky O. Role of marijuana components on the regenerative ability of stem cells. *Cell Biochem Funct.* 2021 Apr;39(3):432–441. doi: 10.1002/cbf.3609. Epub 2020 Dec 21. PMID: 33349985.

9. Habib AM, Okorokov AL, Hill MN, Bras JT, Lee MC, Li S, Gossage SJ, van Drimmelen M, Morena M, Houlden H, Ramirez JD, Bennett DLH, Srivastava D, Cox JJ. Microdeletion in a FAAH pseudogene identified in a patient with high anandamide concentrations and pain insensitivity. *Br J Anaesth.* 2019 Aug;123(2):e249–e253. doi: 10.1016/j.bja.2019.02.019. Epub 2019 Mar 28. PMID: 30929760; PMCID: PMC6676009.

10. Watkins AR. Cannabinoid interactions with ion channels and receptors. *Channels (Austin).* 2019 Dec;13(1):162-167. doi: 10.1080/19336950.2019.1615824. PMID: 31088312; PMCID: PMC6527074.

11. Schuele LL, Schuermann B, Bilkei-Gorzo A, Gorgzadeh S, Zimmer A, Leidmaa E. Regulation of adult neurogenesis by the endocannabinoid-producing enzyme diacylglycerol lipase alpha (DAGLa). *Sci Rep.* 2022 Jan 12;12(1):633. doi: 10.1038/s41598-021-04600-1. PMID: 35022487; PMCID: PMC8755832.

12. Kohler O, Krogh J, Mors O, Benros ME. Inflammation in depression and the potential for anti-inflammatory treatment. *Curr Neuropharmacol.* 2016;14(7):732–42. doi: 10.2174/1570159x14666151208113700. PMID: 27640518; PMCID: PMC5050394.

13. Stein C. Targeting pain and inflammation by peripherally acting opioids. *Front. Pharmacol.* 2013;4:123. doi: 10.3389/fphar.2013.00123.

14. Rios C, Gomes I, Devi LA. Mu opioid and CB1 cannabinoid receptor interactions: reciprocal inhibition of receptor signaling and neuritogenesis. *Br J Pharmacol.* 2006 Jun;148(4):387–95. doi: 10.1038/sj.bjp.0706757. Epub 2006 May 8. PMID: 16682964; PMCID: PMC1751792.

Chapter 12

1. Hasenoehrl C, Taschler U, Storr M, Schicho R. The gastrointestinal tract—a central organ of cannabinoid signaling in health and disease. *Neurogastroenterol Motil.* 2016 Dec;28(12):1765–1780. doi: 10.1111/nmo.12931. Epub 2016 Aug 26. PMID: 27561826; PMCID: PMC5130148.

2. Russo EB. Taming THC: potential cannabis synergy and phytocannabinoid-terpenoid entourage effects. *Br J Pharmacol.* 2011 Aug;163(7):1344–64. doi: 10.1111/j.1476-5381.2011.01238.x. PMID: 21749363; PMCID: PMC3165946.

3. DeFilippis EM, Longman R, Harbus M, et al. Crohn's Disease: evolution, epigenetics, and the emerging role of microbiome-targeted therapies. *Curr Gastroenterol Rep.* 2016;18:13. https://doi.org/10.1007/s11894-016-0487-z.

4. Desborough MJR, Keeling DM. The aspirin story—from willow to wonder drug. *Br J Haematol.* 2017 Jun;177(5):674–683. doi: 10.1111/bjh.14520. Epub 2017 Jan 20. PMID: 28106908.

5. Russo EB. Clinical endocannabinoid deficiency reconsidered: current research supports the theory in migraine, fibromyalgia, irritable bowel, and other treatment-resistant syndromes. *Cannabis Cannabinoid Res.* 2016 Jul 1;1(1):154–165. doi: 10.1089/can.2016.0009. PMID: 28861491; PMCID: PMC5576607.

6. Naftali T, Konikoff FM. Cannabis in inflammatory bowel diseases: from anecdotal use to medicalization? *Isr Med Assoc J.* 2017 Feb;19(2):95–97. PMID: 28457058.

7. Naftali T, Bar-Lev Schleider L, Scklerovsky Benjaminov F, Konikoff FM, Matalon ST, Ringel Y. Cannabis is associated with clinical but not endoscopic remission in ulcerative colitis: A randomized controlled trial. *PLoS One.* 2021 Feb 11;16(2):e0246871. doi: 10.1371/journal.pone.0246871. PMID: 33571293; PMCID: PMC7877751.

8. Round JL, Mazmanian SK. The gut microbiota shapes intestinal immune responses during health and disease. *Nat Rev Immunol.* 2009 May;9(5):313–23. doi: 10.1038/nri2515. Erratum in: *Nat Rev Immunol.* 2009 Aug;9(8):600. PMID: 19343057; PMCID: PMC4095778.

9. Sarmadyan H, Solhi H, Hajimir T, Najarian-Araghi N, Ghaznavi-Rad E. Determination of the antimicrobial effects of hydro-alcoholic extract of cannabis sativa on multiple drug resistant bacteria isolated from nosocomial infections. *Iran. J. Toxicol.* 2014;7:967–972.

10. Al Khoury A, Sleiman R, Atoui A, Hindieh P, Maroun RG, Bailly JD, El Khoury A. Antifungal and anti-aflatoxigenic properties of organs of cannabis sativa L.: relation to phenolic content and antioxidant capacities. *Arch Microbiol.* 2021 Sep;203(7):4485–4492. doi: 10.1007/s00203-021-02444-x. Epub 2021 Jun 18. PMID: 34143269.

11. Lone TA, Lone RA. Extraction of cannabinoids from cannabis sativa L. plant and its potential antimicrobial activity. *Univers. J. Med. Dent.* 2012;1:51–55.

12. Ranganathan M, et al. The effects of cannabinoids on serum cortisol and prolactin in humans. *Psychopharmacology.* 2009;203:737–44.

13. Gugliandolo A, Pollastro F, Grassi G, Bramanti P, Mazzon E. In vitro model of neuroinflammation: efficacy of cannabigerol, a non-psychoactive cannabinoid. *Int J Mol Sci.* 2018 Jul 8;19(7):1992. doi: 10.3390/ijms19071992. PMID: 29986533; PMCID: PMC6073490.

Chapter 13

1. Bíró T, Tóth BI, Haskó G, Paus R, Pacher P. The endocannabinoid system of the skin in health and disease: novel perspectives and therapeutic opportunities. *Trends Pharmacol Sci.* 2009 Aug;30(8):411–20. doi: 10.1016/j.tips.2009.05.004. Epub 2009 Jul 14. PMID: 19608284; PMCID: PMC2757311.

2. Liu C, Qi X, Alhabeil J, Lu H, Zhou Z. Activation of cannabinoid receptors promote periodontal cell adhesion and migration. *J Clin Periodontol.* 2019 Dec;46(12):1264–1272. doi: 10.1111/jcpe.13190. Epub 2019 Oct 22. PMID: 31461164.

3. Karsak M, et al. Attenuation of allergic contact dermatitis through the endocannabinoid system. *Science.* 2007;316:1494–1497.

4. Oláh A, Tóth BI, Borbíró I, Sugawara K, Szöllősi AG, Czifra G, Pál B, Ambrus L, Kloepper J, Camera E, Ludovici M, Picardo M, Voets T, Zouboulis CC, Paus R, Bíró T. Cannabidiol exerts sebostatic and anti-inflammatory effects on human sebocytes. *J Clin Invest.* 2014 Sep;124(9):3713–24. doi: 10.1172/JCI64628. Epub 2014 Jul 25. PMID: 25061872; PMCID: PMC4151231.

5. Karas JA, Wong LJM, Paulin OKA, Mazeh AC, Hussein MH, Li J, Velkov T. The antimicrobial activity of cannabinoids. *Antibiotics (Basel).* 2020 Jul 13;9(7):406. doi: 10.3390/antibiotics9070406. PMID: 32668669; PMCID: PMC7400265.

6. Tüting T, Gaffal E. Regulatory role of cannabinoids for skin barrier functions and cutaneous inflammation, In: Preedy VR, ed. *Handbook of Cannabis and Related Pathologies*. Academic Press; 2017:543–549. doi.org/10.1016/B978 -0-12-800756-3.00067-3.

7. Nguyen LC, Yang D, Nicolaescu V, Best TJ, Gula H, Saxena D, Gabbard JD, Chen SN, Ohtsuki T, Friesen JB, Drayman N, Mohamed A, Dann C, Silva D, Robinson-Mailman L, Valdespino A, Stock L, Suárez E, Jones KA, Azizi SA, Demarco JK, Severson WE, Anderson CD, Millis JM, Dickinson BC, Tay S, Oakes SA, Pauli GF, Palmer KE, National COVID Cohort Collaborative Consortium, Meltzer DO, Randall G, Rosner MR. Cannabidiol inhibits SARS-CoV-2 replication through induction of the host ER stress and innate immune responses. *Sci Adv*. 2022 Feb 25;8(8):eabi6110. doi: 10.1126/sciadv.abi6110. Epub 2022 Feb 23. PMID: 35050692.

8. Mahmud MS, Hossain MS, Ahmed ATMF, Islam MZ, Sarker ME, Islam MR. Antimicrobial and antiviral (SARS-CoV-2) potential of cannabinoids and cannabis sativa: a comprehensive review. *Molecules*. 2021 Nov 28;26(23):7216. doi: 10.3390/molecules26237216. PMID: 34885798; PMCID: PMC8658882.

9. Srivastava BK, et al. Hair growth stimulator property of thienyl substituted pyrazole carboxamide derivatives as a cb1 receptor antagonist with in vivo antiobesity effect. *Bioorg. Med. Chem. Lett.* 2009;19:2546–2550.

Chapter 14

1. Wei D, Lee D, Cox CD, Karsten CA, Peñagarikano O, Geschwind DH, Gall CM, Piomelli D. Endocannabinoid signaling mediates oxytocin-driven social reward. *Proc Natl Acad Sci USA*. 2015 Nov 10;112(45):14084–9. doi: 10.1073 /pnas.1509795112. Epub 2015 Oct 26. PMID: 26504214; PMCID: PMC4653148.

2. Shiff B, Blankstein U, Hussaen J, Jarvi K, Grober E, Lo K, Lajkosz K, Krakowsky Y. The impact of cannabis use on male sexual function: A 10-year, single-center experience. *Can Urol Assoc J*. 2021 Dec;15(12):E652–E657. doi: 10.5489 /cuaj.7185. PMID: 34171210; PMCID: PMC8631840.

3. Lynn BK, López JD, Miller C, Thompson J, Campian EC. The relationship between marijuana use prior to sex and sexual function in women. *Sex Med*. 2019 Jun;7(2):192–197. doi: 10.1016/j.esxm.2019.01.003. Epub 2019 Mar 2. PMID: 30833225; PMCID: PMC6522945.

4. Lynn BK, López JD, Miller C, Thompson J, Campian EC. The relationship between marijuana use prior to sex and sexual function in women. *Sex Med*. 2019 Jun;7(2):192–197. doi: 10.1016/j.esxm.2019.01.003. Epub 2019 Mar 2. PMID: 30833225; PMCID: PMC6522945.

5. Jones RT. Cardiovascular system effects of marijuana. *J Clin Pharmacol.* 2002 Nov;42(S1):58S–63S. doi: 10.1002/j.1552-4604.2002.tb06004.x. PMID: 12412837.

6. Dutton DG, Aron AP. Some evidence for heightened sexual attraction under conditions of high anxiety. *J Pers Soc Psychol.* 1974 Oct;30(4):510–7. doi: 10.1037/h0037031. PMID: 4455773.

7. Fantus RJ, Lokeshwar SD, Kohn TP, Ramasamy R. The effect of tetrahydrocannabinol on testosterone among men in the United States: results from the National Health and Nutrition Examination Survey. *World J Urol.* 2020 Dec;38(12):3275–3282. doi: 10.1007/s00345-020-03110-5. Epub 2020 Feb 17. PMID: 32067074.

8. Allen J, Kenrick D, Linder D, Mccall M. Arousal and attraction: A response-facilitation alternative to misattribution and negative-reinforcement models. *Journal of Personality and Social Psychology.* 1989;57:261–270. 10.1037/0022-3514.57.2.261.

9. Brody S. The relative health benefits of different sexual activities. *J Sex Med.* 2010 Apr;7(4 Pt 1):1336–61. doi: 10.1111/j.1743-6109.2009.01677.x. Epub 2010 Jan 15. PMID: 20088868.

10. Jacobsen SJ, Jacobson DJ, Rohe DE, Girman CJ, Roberts RO, Lieber MM. Frequency of sexual activity and prostatic health: fact or fairy tale? *Urology.* 2003 Feb;61(2):348–53. doi: 10.1016/s0090-4295(02)02265-3. PMID: 12597946.

11. Cabeza de Baca T, Epel ES, Robles TF, Coccia M, Gilbert A, Puterman E, Prather AA. Sexual intimacy in couples is associated with longer telomere length. *Psychoneuroendocrinology.* 2017 Jul;81:46–51. doi: 10.1016/j.psyneuen.2017.03.022. Epub 2017 Mar 25. PMID: 28411413; PMCID: PMC5496682.

12. Payne KS, Mazur DJ, Hotaling JM, Pastuszak AW. Cannabis and male fertility: a systematic review. *J Urol.* 2019 Oct;202(4):674–681. doi: 10.1097/JU.0000000000000248. Epub 2019 Sep 6. PMID: 30916627; PMCID: PMC7385722.

13. Cacciola G, Chianese R, Chioccarelli T, Ciaramella V, Fasano S, Pierantoni R, Meccariello R, Cobellis G. Cannabinoids and reproduction: a lasting and intriguing history. *Pharmaceuticals (Basel).* 2010 Oct 25;3(10):3275–323. doi: 10.3390/ph3103275. PMCID: PMC4034092.

14. Pizzol D, Demurtas J, Stubbs B, Soysal P, Mason C, Isik AT, Solmi M, Smith L, Veronese N. Relationship between cannabis use and erectile dysfunction: a systematic review and meta-analysis. *Am J Mens Health.* 2019 Nov-Dec;13(6):1557988319892464. doi: 10.1177/1557988319892464. PMID: 31795801; PMCID: PMC6893937.

Chapter 15

1. Lukhele ST, Motadi LR. Cannabidiol rather than cannabis sativa extracts inhibit cell growth and induce apoptosis in cervical cancer cells. *BMC Complement Altern Med.* 2016 Sep 1;16(1):335. doi: 10.1186/s12906-016-1280-0. PMID: 27586579; PMCID: PMC5009497.

2. Laezza C, Pagano C, Navarra G, Pastorino O, Proto MC, Fiore D, Piscopo C, Gazzerro P, Bifulco M. The endocannabinoid system: a target for cancer treatment. *Int J Mol Sci.* 2020 Jan 23;21(3):747. doi: 10.3390/ijms21030747. PMID: 31979368; PMCID: PMC7037210.

3. Galanti G, Fisher T, Kventsel I, Shoham J, Gallily R, Mechoulam R, Lavie G, Amariglio N, Rechavi G, Toren A. Delta 9-tetrahydrocannabinol inhibits cell cycle progression by downregulation of E2F1 in human glioblastoma multiforme cells. *Acta Oncol.* 2008;47(6):1062–70. doi: 10.1080/02841860701678787. PMID: 17934890.

4. Borrelli F, Pagano E, Romano B, Panzera S, Maiello F, Coppola D, De Petrocellis L, Buono L, Orlando P, Izzo AA. Colon carcinogenesis is inhibited by the TRPM8 antagonist cannabigerol, a cannabis-derived non-psychotropic cannabinoid. *Carcinogenesis.* 2014 Dec;35(12):2787–97. doi: 10.1093/carcin/bgu205. Epub 2014 Sep 30. PMID: 25269802.

5. Blázquez C, Salazar M, Carracedo A, Lorente M, Egia A, González-Feria L, Haro A, Velasco G, Guzmán M. Cannabinoids inhibit glioma cell invasion by down-regulating matrix metalloproteinase-2 expression. *Cancer Res.* 2008 Mar 15;68(6):1945–52. doi: 10.1158/0008-5472.CAN-07-5176. PMID: 18339876.

6. Mohammadpour F, Ostad SN, Aliebrahimi S, Daman Z. Anti-invasion effects of cannabinoids agonist and antagonist on human breast cancer stem cells. *Iran J Pharm Res.* 2017 Fall;16(4):1479–1486. PMID: 29552056; PMCID: PMC5843309.

7. Horváth B, Mukhopadhyay P, Kechrid M, Patel V, Tanchian G, Wink DA, Gertsch J, Pacher P. β-Caryophyllene ameliorates cisplatin-induced nephrotoxicity in a cannabinoid 2 receptor-dependent manner. *Free Radic Biol Med.* 2012 Apr 15;52(8):1325–33. doi: 10.1016/j.freeradbiomed.2012.01.014. Epub 2012 Jan 31. PMID: 22326488; PMCID: PMC3312970.

8. Ramos JA, Bianco FJ. The role of cannabinoids in prostate cancer: basic science perspective and potential clinical applications. *Indian J Urol.* 2012 Jan;28(1):9–14. doi: 10.4103/0970-1591.94942. PMID: 22557710; PMCID: PMC3339795.

9. Kleckner AS, Kleckner IR, Kamen CS, Tejani MA, Janelsins MC, Morrow GR, Peppone LJ. Opportunities for cannabis in supportive care in cancer. *Ther Adv*

Med Oncol. 2019 Aug 1;11:1758835919866362. doi: 10.1177/1758835919866362. PMID: 31413731; PMCID: PMC6676264.

10. Iwasaki K, Zheng YW, Murata S, Ito H, Nakayama K, Kurokawa T, Sano N, Nowatari T, Villareal MO, Nagano YN, Isoda H, Matsui H, Ohkohchi N. Anticancer effect of linalool via cancer-specific hydroxyl radical generation in human colon cancer. *World J Gastroenterol.* 2016 Nov 28;22(44):9765–9774. doi: 10.3748/wjg.v22.i44.9765. PMID: 27956800; PMCID: PMC5124981.

11. Lu XG, Zhan LB, Feng BA, Qu MY, Yu LH, Xie JH. Inhibition of growth and metastasis of human gastric cancer implanted in nude mice by d-limonene. *World J Gastroenterol.* 2004 Jul 15;10(14):2140–4. doi: 10.3748/wjg.v10.i14 .2140. PMID: 15237454; PMCID: PMC4572353.

Chapter 16

1. Moens K, Higginson IJ, Harding R; EURO IMPACT. Are there differences in the prevalence of palliative care-related problems in people living with advanced cancer and eight non-cancer conditions? A systematic review. *J Pain Symptom Manage.* 2014 Oct;48(4):660–77. doi: 10.1016/j.jpainsymman.2013.11.009. Epub 2014 May 5. PMID: 24801658.

2. Schenker Y, Crowley-Matoka M, Dohan D, Rabow MW, Smith CB, White DB, Chu E, Tiver GA, Einhorn S, Arnold RM. Oncologist factors that influence referrals to subspecialty palliative care clinics. *J Oncol Pract.* 2014 Mar;10(2):e37–44. doi: 10.1200/JOP.2013.001130. Epub 2013 Dec 3. PMID: 24301842; PMCID: PMC3948709.

Index

brain
    cannabis's effect on, 47, 120–123,
        126–127
    and emotional life, 119 (*see also* mental
        health issues)
    fear that cannabis "kills brain cells,"
        161–162
    and headaches, 151, 153–154
    health of, 158, 162 (*see also*
        neurodegenerative diseases)
    interpretation of pain in, 188–189
    and seizures, 172–173
    and sexual relations, 233
brain cancer, 244
breastfeeding, 111
bud site, 7
butin, 22

C

cadinene, 15
Cameron, Jo, 37, 186
camphene, 15
camphor, 15
cancer and cancer therapy symptoms,
    242–256
    cannabis treatment for, 244–246
    dosages in cannabis treatment for,
        249–251
    making decisions about diagnosis,
        244
    making decisions about using cannabis,
        257
    pretreating cancer after diagnosis, 253
    prostate cancer, 246
    regimens for cancer treatment, 248–252
    regimens for treating symptoms,
        247–248
    traditional treatments for, 243, 248,
        252, 254, 255
cannabinoids, 7–13
    boiling points for, 85–89
    CBD, 9–10 (*see also* CBD [cannabidiol])
    as conduit across separate body systems,
        38

    extracting, 85
    men's prolonged exposure to, 236
    synergy of terpenes, flavonoids, and,
        202
    THC, 9–10 (*see also* THC
        [tetrahydrocannabinol])
    types and uses of, 10–11 (*see also*
        individual types)
cannabis
    aging of, 29
    benefits of, xii
    decarboxylating, 83–84
    effects of (*see* using cannabis)
    information and education about, xi,
        xiv–xv
    interactions among other therapies and,
        107, 108
    legalization of, xi
    medical guidance model for, xii–xviii
    pharmacies for, xviii
    science on, xiii–xiv (*see also* research on
        cannabis)
    side effects of, xiii
    smoking, 58–59
    typical experiences with, 29–31
    used a coping mechanism, 103
    use of term, 5
cannabis as medicine, xi–xviii, 37–38,
    265–266. *see also* using cannabis
    in early twentieth century, 32–33
    guided cannabis medical practice,
        xii–xviii (*see also* guided cannabis
        journey)
    treatment protocol model changed
        by, xii–xiii (*see also specific health
        issues*)
cannabis butter, 92–93, 250
cannabis plant, 3–29
    botany of, 6–7
    chemical components in, 4–5, 7–28
    gene pools of, 4, 6
    increased THC in, 30
    making products from, 28–29 (*see also*
        cannabis products)

290 Index

F

farnesene, 17
fecal incontinence, 207
feedback inhibition, 187–188
fenchol, 17
fertility, 234–235
fisetin, 23
flavonoids, 7, 21–28
  benefits of, 21
  extracting, 85
  for mental health issues, 131
  for skin conditions, 219
  synergy of cannabinoids, terpenes, and, 202
  types and uses of, 21–28 (see also individual types)
  upgrading flowers with, 84
flower derivatives, inhalation options for, 58–62
flowers, 7
  decarboxylating, 83–84
  inhalation options for, 58–62
  from online marketplaces, 252
  upgrading, 84
focal seizures, 172
follicular lymphoma, 254
food(s)
  and gastrological issues, 215
  high in terpenes, 14
  upgrading, 98–100
forgetfulness, 103, 230
fustin, 23

G

galangin, 23
gamma-aminobutyric acid (GABA), 175–176
gas/bloating, 207
gastroesophageal reflux disease (GERD), 207–208, 213
gastrological (GI) issues, 201–215
  appetite and cannabis, 208–209
  with cancer, 247
  cannabis and the microbiome, 205

cannabis for treating inflammation and infection, 109, 203–205
cannabis regimens for, 213–215
causes of, 202
CBG for, 211–212
and endocannabinoid deficiency, 203
and food choices, 215
mental distress causing stomach upset, 209–211
mind-gut connection, 98
and oral products, 212–213
physiological, addressing, 205–208
traditional medications for, 213
gateway drug, cannabis as, 47
gender identification, 230
generalized seizures, 172–173
genistein, 24
genistin, 24
genital sensation, reduced, 238
genkwanin, 24
geraldol, 24
geraniol, 17
GERD (gastroesophageal reflux disease), 207–208, 213
GI issues. see gastrological issues
ginkgetin, 24
glabridin, 24
glycitein, 24
glycitin, 24
goals for health, 111
gossypetin, 24
G protein-lined receptors, 34
grand mal seizures, 173
guaiol, 17
guided cannabis journey, 97–115
  adapting physical space, 105
  adopting exercise program, 101–102
  and cannabis used a coping mechanism, 103
  control in, 44–45
  current health status information, 108–109
  effects of cannabis in (see using cannabis)

pain (*continued*)
    with terminal illnesses, 260
    transmission of signaling from a source,
        187–188
    types of, 182
palliation, 243
palliative care, 257, 259. *see also* end-of-life
    plan
pancreatic cancer, 244
para-cymene, 19
paranoia, 42, 43, 122
Parkinson's disease, 166–169
    cannabis treatment regimens for,
        170–171
    present understanding of, 158–159
    traditional medications for, 168–169
paroxysmal hemicrania, 150
patches
    during cancer treatment, 247
    in end-of-life care, 260
    optimal dosages of, 71–72
    for physical pain, 191, 198
    for seizures, 177
    for skin conditions, 225, 226
patuletin, 26
peacefulness, using cannabis for, 38–40
peristalsis, 205
personalized treatment, xiii, xiv, xix
pharmaceuticals. *see also* over-the-counter
    (OTC) pharmaceuticals; prescription
    medications
    cannabis therapies vs., 37–38, 41
    in current medical model, 109
    not using cannabis to replace, 107–108
    for pain management, 187
    safety profiles for, 44
α-phellandrene, 20
phloretin, 26
phloridzin, 27
physical aspects of sex, 231–233
physical pain, 181–200. *see also* headaches;
    pain
    brain's interpretation of, 188–189
    cannabis regimens for, 195–198
    cannabis's effect on, 182–190

cannabis vs. other treatments for,
        192–195
    damage from everyday life, 185
    defining, 182
    facets of, 187
    gastrointestinal, 201
    having an identity of, 190
    inflammation reduction, 183–184
    memory of, 189
    mental distraction from, 186
    mobility improvement, 183
    tissue healing, 184–185
    transmission of pain signaling from a
        source, 187–188
physical space, adapting, 105
phytocannabinoids, 33
phytol, 19
pills, 93, 170, 250
α-pinene, 20
β-pinene, 21
pinocembrin, 27
placebo effect, 37, 39
pleasant side effects, 43–44
pleasure, 235
polypharmacy, 109
poncirin, 27
population-based medicine, xii–xiii
post-traumatic stress disorder (PTSD),
    39–40, 78, 126–127, 189
pregnancy, 111
prescription medications. *see also*
    pharmaceuticals
    adding cannabis to, 132, 157
    cannabis, 62, 64, 163, 176–177
    enhancing effectiveness of, 41, 143
    evaluating existing medications, 106–108
    interactions among, xiii
    interactions among other therapies and,
        106–107
proliferation, of cancer cells, 245
prostate cancer, 233, 246
psoriasis, 221
psychoactive (term), 8
PTSD. *see* post-traumatic stress disorder
pulegone, 19

About the Author

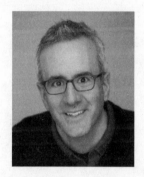

Benjamin Caplan, MD, is a licensed, board-certified doctor of family medicine. He is a graduate of Williams College and completed his medical degree at Tufts University School of Medicine and residency in family medicine at the Boston Medical Center. Dr. Caplan has served as an investigator for multiple pharmaceutical research studies and has published in leading medical journals, including the *New England Journal of Medicine*. He has served as a formal supervisor of a Harvard Medical School fellow of geriatric medicine and supervises several medical school students and undergraduates. He is the founder and chief medical officer of CED Clinic, EO Care, Inc., and CED Foundation, three industry-leading patient care and digital education organizations. For more information, visit www.caplancannabis.com.